YOUR GUT IS YOUR SECOND BRAIN

THE SCIENCE-BACKED PLAN TO OPTIMIZE DIGESTIVE HEALTH, BALANCE THE MICROBIOME, BOOST IMMUNITY, AND SUPPORT WEIGHT LOSS FOR A HAPPIER HEALTHIER YOU

BY
ORLANDO WRIGHT

© **2025** by Cheerful Sprouts LLC

All rights reserved. No part of this book may be reproduced in any form or by any electronic or mechanical means, including information storage and retrieval systems, without permission in writing from the author.

The content of this book is for general informational purposes only. Each person's physical, emotional, and spiritual condition is unique. The instruction in this book is not meant to be used, nor should it be used, to diagnose or treat any medical condition or to replace the services of your physician or other healthcare provider. The advice and strategies contained in the book may not be suitable for all readers. Please consult your healthcare provider for any questions that you may have about your own medical situation. Neither the author, publisher, nor any of their employees or representatives guarantees the accuracy of information in this book or its usefulness to a particular reader, nor are they responsible for any damage or negative consequence that may result from any treatment, action taken, or inaction by any person reading or following the information in this book.

ISBN: 978-1-968170-01-1

Printed in the United States of America

TABLE OF CONTENTS

PREFACE   1

INTRODUCTION   2

CHAPTER 1 WHAT IS THE GUT AND THE GUT'S ECOSYSTEM?   4

    THE DIGESTIVE PROCESS EXPLAINED   4
    THE MICROBIOME: YOUR INNER ECOSYSTEM   8
    GOOD BACTERIA VS. BAD BACTERIA: FINDING BALANCE   12

CHAPTER 2 YOUR GUT AND YOUR BODY   15

    MAPPING THE GUT-BRAIN CONNECTION   15
    MENTAL HEALTH AND THE GUT   19
    HOW GUT HEALTH INFLUENCES IMMUNITY   21
    THE ROLE OF GUT FLORA IN METABOLISM   23
    GUT HEALTH AND HORMONAL BALANCE   25
    HOW GUT HEALTH INFLUENCES WEIGHT MANAGEMENT   27

CHAPTER 3 COMMON GUT ISSUES AND THEIR ROOTS   30

    IBS AND BEYOND: COMMON DIGESTIVE DISORDERS   30
    UNPACKING FOOD INTOLERANCES AND ALLERGIES   32
    LEAKY GUT: SEPARATING FACT FROM FICTION   34
    UNDERSTANDING INFLAMMATION IN THE GUT   36
    STRESS AND ITS DIRECT IMPACT ON DIGESTION   37
    THE AGE-RELATED DIGESTIVE DECLINE   39

CHAPTER 4 GUT HEALTH ACROSS THE LIFESPAN   42

    NURTURING GUT HEALTH IN CHILDREN:
    BUILDING IMMUNITY AND WELLNESS   42
    MANAGING GUT ISSUES DURING ADOLESCENCE   44
    GUT HEALTH STRATEGIES FOR YOUNG ADULTS   46
    ADAPTING TO MIDLIFE CHANGES IN GUT FUNCTION   48
    SUPPORTING DIGESTIVE HEALTH IN OLDER ADULTS   50
    FAMILY FRIENDLY GUT HEALTH PRACTICES   52

CHAPTER 5 NUTRITION: THE CORNERSTONE OF GUT HEALTH   54

    PROBIOTICS 101: CHOOSING THE RIGHT STRAINS   54
    THE PREBIOTIC POWER: FUEL FOR YOUR MICROBES   59
    DESIGNING A GUT-FRIENDLY PLATE   63
    FERMENTED FOODS: NATURAL PROBIOTICS   65
    THE ANTI-INFLAMMATORY DIET: A GUT HEALTH ALLY   67
    CRAFTING FAMILY-FRIENDLY GUT HEALTH RECIPES   69

CHAPTER 6 PERSONALIZED GUT HEALTH PROTOCOLS 72

- Crafting a Personalized Gut Health Plan — 72
- Tailoring Your Diet to Combat IBS — 75
- Supporting Gut Health in Aging Adults — 77
- Addressing Children's Gut Health Needs — 81
- Managing Food Sensitivities with Precision — 82
- Troubleshooting Common Gut Health Challenges — 84
- Building a Support System for Your Gut Health Journey — 86

CHAPTER 7 THE FOUR-WEEK PROTOCOL: A ROADMAP TO GUT HEALTH EXPANDED 88

- Week 1: Cleansing and Resetting Your Gut — 88
- Week 2: Reintroducing Nutrients with Purpose — 94
- Week 3 Meal Plan: Cultivating Diversity — 103
- Week 4: Strengthening Immunity and Longevity — 106
- The Role of Supplements: When and How to Use Them — 112
- Tracking Progress: Assessing Your Gut Health Journey — 113

CHAPTER 8 LIFESTYLE AND THE GUT HEALTH CONNECTION 114

- How Hydration Affects Digestion — 114
- The Sleep-Digestion Connection — 115
- Stress Management Techniques for Better Gut Health — 117
- The Role of Physical Activity in Digestion — 119
- Digital Detox: Limiting Screen Time for Better Sleep — 123
- Breathing Techniques to Enhance Gut Function — 125

CHAPTER 9 IMPLEMENTING CHANGES AND SUSTAINING SUCCESS 127

- Building a Support System for Gut Health — 127
- Staying Motivated: Tracking Your Progress — 130
- Overcoming Setbacks: What to Do When Symptoms Persist — 132
- Celebrating Small Wins in Gut Health — 133
- Engaging with the Gut Health Community — 135
- The Future of Gut Health: Embracing Science and Technology — 138

CONCLUSION 140

APPENDIX I: LEARNING TO BREATHE 143

APPENDIX II: LEARNING TO MEDITATE 146

REFERENCES 149

PREFACE

Let me start with a story. A few years ago, I found myself battling constant bloating and discomfort. No matter what I ate, my gut seemed to rebel. I tried ignoring it at first, thinking it was just a phase, temporary, and if I could find out which foods were causing it, I could just eliminate them. But that didn't bring any relief, and before I realized what was happening, those minor annoyances turned into more serious issues—irritable bowel syndrome, fatigue, and even mood swings. It was as if my body was speaking a language I couldn't understand, and I had to learn to listen.

What I discovered as I delved into the world of gut health was that this complex network of microbes and neural pathways plays a pivotal role in regulating our immune system, metabolism, and even our mental health. This was the key I began with to heal my gut.

However, I also realized that the path to gut healing was not a one-size-fits-all approach. The conflicting advice and inconsistent results I had experienced were a testament to the need for a personalized, science-backed plan. And that is why I wrote this book. When I found what worked for me and why, I knew that I wanted to share this knowledge with others who were struggling, offering them a roadmap to navigate the often-confusing landscape of gut health.

The primary goal here is straightforward: to offer you a science-backed plan to optimize your digestive health. We'll explore how to balance your microbiome, boost your immunity, and support weight loss.

INTRODUCTION

Why is gut health so important, you might wonder? Our gut is often called the "second brain." This isn't just a catchy phrase. It's rooted in science. The gut-brain axis is a complex communication network linking our digestive system with our brain. This connection influences our mood, immune system, and overall health. It might surprise you to learn that around 70% of our immune cells reside in the gut. Moreover, the gut produces about 90% of our body's serotonin, a key neurotransmitter that regulates mood. These facts underscore the significant role the gut plays in our health.

In this book, "Your Gut Is Your Second Brain", I introduce a four-week protocol designed to bring about what I call a "smart gut". This program is not just about what you eat, but how you live. Over the course of four weeks, you'll learn how to make changes that are sustainable and impactful. We'll dive into meal plans and actionable tips that make the science practical and, most importantly, achievable. Through a holistic approach that prioritizes natural solutions and food-based interventions, we will address the root causes of digestive issues and pave the way for lasting wellness.

Throughout these pages, you will discover:

- The intricate relationship between your gut microbiome and overall health

- The impact of stress, sleep, and lifestyle factors on gut function

- Nourishing recipes and meal plans to support digestive healing

- Targeted supplements and probiotics to restore balance

- A 4-week gut healing protocol to jumpstart your journey

So, who is this book for? If you're struggling with digestive issues like bloating or IBS, this book is for you. If you're a parent wanting to establish healthy eating habits for your family, you'll find valuable insights here. Health professionals will also discover science-backed information that can aid their practice. And if you're simply someone curious about the connection between gut health and overall well-being, you're in the right place.

It's about food, yes, but it's also about a lifestyle that enables you to understand how digestion, absorption, and homeostasis work; how the brain and gut are connected, and how, in conjunction with detoxifying your body, you can pave the way for better thinking, less pain, fewer digestive issues, and natural energy.

So, I invite you to join me on this enlightening path to optimal health. Together, we will unravel the mysteries of the gut, armed with the latest scientific insights and a compassionate, empowering approach. Let us celebrate the incredible resilience of our bodies and embark on a journey that will transform your relationship with food, your gut, and your overall well-being. Your gut is your second brain, and it holds the key to unlocking a vibrant, thriving, energetic life. Let's begin this adventure together, one mindful step at a time.

CHAPTER 1
WHAT IS THE GUT AND THE GUT'S ECOSYSTEM?

There was a time, not too long ago, when I found myself in a café, sipping on a soothing herbal tea, while a friend animatedly recounted her recent health journey. She spoke of newfound energy, a clearer mind, and the disappearance of long-ailing digestive woes. Her transformation seemed almost magical, yet deeply grounded in something as fundamental as gut health. I listened, intrigued, as she described how understanding the gut's role in our body had changed everything. That conversation lingered with me, prompting a deeper exploration into what truly goes on within us when we eat, absorb, and live. This chapter aims to demystify that journey, to take you on a tour of the gut's incredible ecosystem, and to lay the groundwork for appreciating its profound influence on our overall health.

The Digestive Process Explained

The Mouth

The digestive process is an extraordinary symphony of actions and reactions, all beginning the moment food enters your mouth. As you take that first bite, your teeth work diligently, breaking down the food into smaller, more manageable pieces. Simultaneously, your salivary glands spring into action, secreting enzymes like amylase that initiate the breakdown of carbohydrates.

This isn't just about chewing; it's the first crucial step in digestion, setting the stage for everything that follows. The act of eating becomes a sensory experience, as flavors are released and savored, signaling to your brain that nourishment is on its way. This sensory interaction is more than pleasurable; it's a vital part of digestion, as your brain sends signals to the rest of your digestive system to prepare for the incoming task.

The Esophagus

Once the food is adequately chewed and mixed with saliva, it forms a bolus, a small, soft mass ready to journey down the esophagus. The esophagus, a muscular tube, plays a critical role in guiding this bolus toward the stomach. This movement isn't passive; it's an active process known as peristalsis, where rhythmic, wave-like contractions of the esophageal muscles propel the food downward. This is where the magic of the digestive system begins to unfold, as each part of the process seamlessly transitions into the next, with every organ playing its part in harmony. You can trust that your body knows precisely what to do, even if you aren't consciously aware of it.

The Stomach

As the bolus reaches the stomach, it encounters an environment specifically designed for its breakdown. The stomach, a muscular organ, churns the food with powerful acids and enzymes such as pepsin. These substances work together to transform the solid bolus into a semi-liquid state known as chyme. This is a crucial transformation, as the stomach's acidic environment (hydrochloric acid) is essential for breaking down proteins and killing any harmful bacteria that may have been ingested with the food. The process is both mechanical and chemical, with the stomach's muscular walls contracting to mix the chyme thoroughly. This stage of digestion is intense, as the stomach's lining protects itself from its own acidic environment, a testament to the body's remarkable ability to maintain balance.

The stomach also has the critical job of regulating the release of chyme into the small intestine. This is done with incredible precision, ensuring that the small intestine receives the chyme in manageable amounts that it can effectively process. The pyloric sphincter, a muscular valve at the stomach's exit, plays a crucial role in this regulation, opening and closing to allow small amounts of chyme to pass through. This controlled release is vital, as it ensures that the small intestine, with its vast array of enzymes and absorptive surfaces, can efficiently continue the digestive process. As the chyme enters the small intestine, it encounters a new environment, where absorption and further breakdown of nutrients take place.

The Small Intestine

The small intestine is a marvel of biological engineering, with its extensive surface area lined with villi and microvilli that maximize nutrient absorption. Here, enzymes from the pancreas and bile from the liver continue the breakdown of carbohydrates, proteins, and fats, allowing the nutrients to be absorbed into the bloodstream. This process is not only about breaking down food but also about extracting every possible nutrient to fuel your body's needs. The small intestine's design is optimal for this task, with its twenty-foot-long, coiled structure providing ample time and space for digestion and absorption.

Where does it go from there? The large intestine is the final destination for any waste that is not utilized by the body.

Throughout this process, the body's efficiency and adaptability shine. The digestive system is a testament to the intricate design and function of the human body, working tirelessly to transform food into the energy and building blocks needed to sustain life. It's a reminder of the importance of caring for this system, as its health is directly linked to your overall well-being. Understanding this process is the first step in appreciating the role your gut plays in maintaining health and vitality.

Recap (1)

The gastrointestinal tract is made up of all the hollow organs from the mouth to the colon.

- Mouth
- Esophagus
- Stomach
- Small Intestine
- Large Intestine
- Colon

Solid organs contribute and together with the hollow organs, they make up what we call the gut.

- Liver
- Pancreas
- Gallbladder

Reflective Exercise: Mindful Eating Practice

Take a moment during your next meal to consciously engage with the digestive process. Focus on the flavors, textures, and aromas of your food. Chew slowly, paying attention to the sensation of each bite. Consider the journey your food takes as it moves from your mouth to your stomach and beyond. Sit up straight and relax your stomach and abdomen so food can pass unobstructed. Reflect on how mindful eating can enhance your appreciation of the digestive process and contribute to better gut health. This practice not only fosters a deeper connection with your body's natural rhythms but also encourages a more intentional approach to nourishment.

The Microbiome: Your Inner Ecosystem

When I first heard about the microbiome, it was as if I had stumbled upon a hidden world, teeming with life, right inside of me. Imagine an intricate, bustling metropolis, populated by trillions of microorganisms—bacteria, viruses, fungi—all coexisting in what is designed to be a delicate balance—all the organisms that live within us and interact with each other. This is the microbiome, a microscopic community residing predominantly in your gut, orchestrating a symphony of biological processes that keep you thriving. It's awe-inspiring when you think about it: a living ecosystem within us, influencing nearly every aspect of our health. Each microorganism has a role, contributing to the harmony that is crucial for our well-being. In this microscopic universe, bacteria are the stars, with countless species each performing unique functions. These functions range from aiding digestion to synthesizing vital nutrients. Some bacteria break down complex carbohydrates, transforming them into short-chain fatty acids that nourish your gut lining and support immune function. Others produce essential vitamins, like Vitamin K and various B vitamins, ensuring your body has the tools it needs to function optimally. It's a finely-tuned machine, where each part is indispensable, and the whole is greater than the sum of its parts.

Microbiome Diversity: Why Variety is Key

Diversity within the microbiome acts as a fortress, enhancing our body's resistance to diseases and optimizing metabolic processes. Imagine your gut as a vibrant ecosystem where each microbe plays a unique role. A diverse microbiome can fend off pathogens more effectively and ensure efficient nutrient processing. This variety mirrors a well-tended garden, where different plants contribute to a thriving environment, working synchronistically within the ecosystem.

When this variety shrinks, imbalances arise, allowing harmful bacteria to take hold, potentially leading to health issues such as inflammatory bowel disease or obesity. Thus, maintaining diversity becomes critical, not just for gut health but for overall resilience against diseases.

Dietary habits are significant influencers of microbiome diversity. A varied diet introduces a range of nutrients and fibers that feed different microbial species. This variety ensures no single bacterial type dominates, which could lead to an imbalance. Environmental factors also play a role; exposure to different microorganisms through soil or pet interactions can enrich microbial diversity. Urban environments often limit microbial exposure compared to rural settings, where interaction with nature is more frequent. The interplay of these factors highlights the need for conscious lifestyle choices that encourage diversity and, by extension, robust health.

Enhancing microbiome diversity is achievable through simple, mindful actions. Including fermented foods like kefir or kimchi introduces beneficial bacteria into your diet. Rotating your food choices can also prevent the dominance of any single microbial type. For example, replacing your usual grain with quinoa or buckwheat offers new fibers and nutrients for different bacteria. Seasonal eating further supports diversity, as seasonal foods align more closely with natural cycles and provide varied microbial substrates throughout the year. Such strategies aren't just about what you eat but how you choose to engage with the world.

Real-life transformations underscore the power of a diverse microbiome. Consider the case of a middle-aged woman struggling with chronic digestive discomfort and lethargy. By making small changes—incorporating more plant-based foods, experimenting with new grains, and embracing fermented products—she experienced significant improvements in her energy levels and digestion.

Her story echoes many others who have found relief and vitality by nurturing their microbiome's diversity. These personal accounts serve as powerful reminders of the tangible benefits that come from prioritizing gut health.

Reflecting on these stories, it's clear that investing in microbiome diversity offers numerous rewards. Beyond immediate digestive relief, it enhances immunity and supports metabolic processes, paving the way for long-term health benefits. This approach isn't about drastic changes but small, sustainable adjustments that align with your body's natural rhythms. By fostering a diverse microbial ecosystem within your gut, you lay the foundation for a healthier, more resilient life.

What you consume directly influences which bacteria thrive and which diminish.

- Fiber-rich foods, for instance, feed beneficial bacteria, promoting a healthy, diverse microbiome. Conversely, a diet high in industrially processed foods and sugars can encourage the growth of harmful bacteria, upsetting the balance and potentially leading to toxic build-up. (2)

- Antibiotics, while life-saving, can also have a profound impact, often wiping out beneficial bacteria along with the harmful ones. This disruption can take time to correct, highlighting the importance of mindful antibiotic use. Please make sure you are not taking antibiotics for viral infections. Antibiotics are designed for bacterial infections.

- Lifestyle choices, such as stress management, exercise, and sleep, also affect your microbiome. Chronic stress, for example, can alter the gut environment, affecting its microbial inhabitants.

- Regular physical activity, on the other hand, has been shown to enhance microbial diversity, promoting a more robust microbiome.

- Sleep, too, plays a part; irregular sleep patterns can disrupt gut health, leading to imbalance.

It's clear that caring for your microbiome requires a holistic approach, considering not just diet but the entirety of your lifestyle.

Reflective Exercise: Consider Your Microbiome

Take a moment to reflect on your daily habits. Consider your diet, stress levels, and lifestyle choices. Do you overeat or eat when you're not hungry? Do you sacrifice sleep for after-hours fun more often than you should? Do you drink alcohol regularly? These are all factors that can be influencing your microbiome.

Write down three changes you could make to support a healthier balance. For example:

- Adding more fiber-rich foods to your meals.

- Finding ways to reduce stress.

- Reading labels to find out exactly what's in your food.

- Creating a better sleep environment.

- Eating slowly to give your stomach time to digest.

- Eliminating at least one food you know is bad for you.

These small, mindful adjustments can have a significant impact on your inner ecosystem and, consequently, your overall health. Understanding and nurturing your microbiome is not just about improving digestion; it's about enhancing your entire well-being, providing your body with the resilience it needs to thrive.

Good Bacteria vs. Bad Bacteria: Finding Balance

In the vast and intricate world of your gut, beneficial bacteria play a pivotal role, serving as unsung heroes of your health. Among them, the Lactobacillus and Bifidobacterium strains are particularly notable. They are the champions of your digestive system, tirelessly working to maintain balance. These good bacteria facilitate the breakdown of food, assist in the absorption of nutrients, and produce essential vitamins. They also play a crucial role in maintaining the integrity of the gut lining, acting as a formidable barrier against the onslaught of pathogens. By occupying space and consuming resources, they prevent harmful bacteria from gaining a foothold and wreaking havoc. Their presence is like having a dedicated team of guardians, vigilantly protecting your gut's ecosystem.

Yet, the balance between these beneficial bacteria and their harmful counterparts is delicate. When pathogenic bacteria multiply unchecked, which can happen due to any of the reasons mentioned, they disrupt this balance, often with detrimental effects. Clostridium difficile, for instance, is a notorious pathogen that can cause severe intestinal infections, especially after antibiotic use when defences are low. These infections can lead to inflammation, diarrhea, and more severe complications if not addressed promptly.

Pathogen-induced inflammation arises when bad bacteria proliferate. This inflammation can lead to discomfort and, over time, contribute to chronic conditions such as inflammatory bowel disease. The presence of harmful bacteria can also compromise your immune system, making it more challenging to fend off other infections.

Achieving and maintaining a healthy balance in your gut requires conscious effort and lifestyle changes. One of the most significant and effective ways to promote the growth of beneficial bacteria is through dietary adjustments.

- Incorporating fiber-rich foods, such as fruits, vegetables, and whole grains, into your meals provides the nourishment that good bacteria thrive on. These foods are rich in prebiotics, non-digestible fibers that feed beneficial bacteria, promoting their growth and activity.

- Reducing or eliminating the intake of processed sugar is equally important, as high sugar levels can encourage the growth of harmful bacteria.

- A study (3) done by UCSF showed that eating raw foods or foods as close to their natural state as possible will contribute to your intake of prebiotics, digestive enzymes, phytochemicals, and other nutrients that aid in digestion and the proliferation of good bacteria that protect your gut and your health.

By choosing a diet rich in whole foods, you not only support your gut health but also enhance your overall well-being.

Probiotics, which are live microorganisms that confer health benefits when consumed, can also be a valuable tool in maintaining gut balance. Available in fermented foods like yogurt, kefir, and sauerkraut, as well as in supplement form, probiotics introduce beneficial bacteria directly into your gut. They can help restore balance, particularly after disruptions such as antibiotic treatments. However, not all probiotics are created equal. It's important to choose probiotic strains that are well-researched and suited to your specific needs. Lactobacillus and Bifidobacterium, for example, have been extensively studied and are known for their health-promoting properties.

Prebiotics, on the other hand, provide the nourishment that allows these probiotics to flourish. Found in foods like garlic, onions, and bananas, prebiotics are essential for sustaining a healthy microbiome. They act as food for the good bacteria, ensuring that they remain active and effective. By incorporating both probiotics and prebiotics into your diet, you can create a symbiotic relationship where both thrive, leading to improved gut health. This approach is not about quick fixes but about fostering an environment where beneficial bacteria can flourish naturally.

Maintaining a healthy gut balance is more than just a dietary endeavor; it's a holistic lifestyle choice. Regular physical activity, adequate sleep, and stress management are all crucial components. Exercise has been shown to increase microbial diversity, which is a marker of a healthy gut. Sleep, often overlooked, is essential for the repair and maintenance of bodily functions, including those of the gut. Chronic stress, conversely, can disrupt the gut-brain axis, leading to imbalances and digestive issues. By integrating these elements into your life, you support not only your gut health but your overall well-being.

Reflect on the choices you make daily. How do they impact your gut's delicate balance? Consider the foods you eat, the stress you manage or think you're managing, and the rest you allow yourself. These factors collectively contribute to the state of your microbiome. If you find areas in need of change, make adjustments gradually. Introduce more fiber-rich foods, explore the world of fermented products, and seek ways to reduce stress. The journey towards optimal gut health is ongoing and requires patience and perseverance.

In the grand scheme of things, your gut is a microcosm of life—a delicate ecosystem where balance is paramount. The interplay between good and bad bacteria is a dance, one that requires careful attention and nurturing. By understanding the roles these microorganisms play, you empower yourself to make informed decisions that support this balance. Your gut health is a reflection of your lifestyle choices, and with a thoughtful approach, you can cultivate an environment where beneficial bacteria thrive, pathogens are kept at bay, and your overall health flourishes. Embrace this knowledge, and let it guide you toward a healthier, more balanced life.

CHAPTER 2
YOUR GUT AND YOUR BODY

Mapping the Gut-Brain Connection

The gut-brain axis, a fascinating and complex communication network, connects our enteric nervous system with the central nervous system. Imagine it as a bustling highway of information, where messages continually travel between the gut and brain. This bidirectional system uses pathways like the vagus nerve, a critical conduit that contains 75% of your parasympathetic nervous system's nerve fibers, (4) to relay signals between the brain, heart, and digestive system. It also involves neurotransmitters produced in the gut itself. Serotonin, often dubbed the "feel-good" neurotransmitter, is significantly produced in the gut, influencing mood and emotional well-being. This intricate connection means our digestive health directly affects our mental state, and vice versa, creating an interconnectedness that underscores the importance of maintaining a balanced gut.

This relationship has profound psychological implications. You might notice that after a stressful day, your stomach feels off. You feel "sick to your stomach." Stress can exacerbate digestive issues by disrupting the gut-brain communication. Similarly, poor gut health can lead to heightened anxiety or even depression. The phenomenon is more common than you might think. Many people live in this cycle of stress and digestive discomfort without realizing the two are linked. Studies (5) have shown that enhancing gut health can lead to reduced levels of stress and anxiety, thus a healthier gut contributes not only to a clearer mind and a more stable mood but to a more harmonious life.

Research supports this connection. Clinical trials have explored how alterations in gut bacteria can impact psychological conditions. For instance, one study (6) found that patients who consumed certain probiotics reported decreased levels of anxiety and improved mood markers compared to those who didn't (Mayer et al., 2015). These findings suggest that nurturing a healthy gut microbiome can play a critical role in supporting mental health. The potential of using probiotics to manage not only physical ailments but also psychological ones opens new avenues for holistic health approaches. Such insights encourage us to view our digestive system as integral to mental well-being.

To optimize the gut-brain axis, practical steps can be taken. Mindfulness practices offer a powerful tool for calming the mind and soothing the gut. Engaging in activities like meditation or yoga helps reduce stress, fostering a healthier digestive environment. Diet plays a crucial role too. Incorporating foods rich in omega-3 fatty acids, such as fatty fish, can support brain health while promoting a balanced gut microbiome. Fermented foods like kombucha, sugar-free yogurt or naturally fermented sauerkraut introduce beneficial bacteria that enhance gut function and, consequently, mental clarity.

Interactive Element: Mindfulness Practice

Take five minutes each day to focus on your breathing. Find a quiet space, sit comfortably, and close your eyes. Inhale deeply through your nose, hold for a moment, then exhale slowly through your mouth. As you breathe, visualize stress leaving your body with each exhale. This simple practice can ease tension in both your mind and digestive system. (See Appendix I: Learning to Breathe).

Additionally, it's important to recognize how lifestyle choices impact this axis. Exercise not only benefits physical health but also stimulates the production of endorphins, improving mood and reducing stress levels. Regular physical activity supports gut motility and aids in maintaining a healthy weight, which is linked to better mental health outcomes.

Dietary adjustments also contribute significantly to this balance. Reducing processed foods and sugar intake while increasing fiber consumption can create a more favorable environment for beneficial gut bacteria. These bacteria produce short-chain fatty acids that nourish intestinal cells and communicate with the brain to positively influence mood. Opt for natural sweeteners like honey or stevia in limited amounts and include whole, unprocessed grains in your meals for sustained energy without the inflammatory downsides of refined sugars and flours. Such mindful choices can have transformative effects on mental health, paving the way for greater emotional resilience and clarity.

Additionally, different types of foods take more or less time to digest, so proper food combining is critical. For example, combining proteins and starches in one meal may cause bloating and gas, as well as weight gain. Combining protein and sugar, particularly under high heat, can accelerate aging by slowing down cell activity through Advanced Glycation End Products, putting you at risk for chronic disease. (7)

The following table give you an idea of which foods work best together and which combinations to avoid. (8)

Category	Mixing Guidelines	Examples
Vegetables	Mixes with everything except fruit	Bell peppers, Brussels sprouts, Green beans, Broccoli, Asparagus, Cabbage, Kale, Onions, Radish, Squash, Eggplant
Protein	Mixes with veggies & neutrals	Milk, Fish, Eggs, Cheese
Starches	Mixes with veggies and neutrals	Yams, Potatoes, Sweet potatoes, Rice, Peas, Water chestnuts, Plantains, Legumes, Grains
Fruit	Eat alone, except melons	Sweet fruits, Sub-acid fruits, Acid fruits
Melon	Do not combine with other foods	Cantaloupe, Watermelon, Honeydew
Neutral	Mixes with everything except fruit	Vegetables (repeated here for neutral behavior), Lemons, Limes, Fats & oils, Olives, Avocados, Herbs & spices, Nuts, Seeds
Other Neutrals	Same as above	Plain yogurt, Stevia, Dark chocolate (70%+), Raw honey, Pure maple syrup, Fermented foods, Coconut water, Coconut milk, Buttermilk

Engaging with recent scientific findings allows us to appreciate how interconnected our bodies truly are. The insights gained from studying the gut-brain axis highlight the importance of integrative approaches to health—approaches that consider both physical and mental dimensions. By embracing these strategies, we take steps toward not only enhancing digestive health but also enriching our emotional resilience.

Mental Health and the Gut

In my quest to understand the interconnectedness of gut health and mental well-being, I discovered a fascinating truth: your gut is a powerhouse for serotonin production. Serotonin, often referred to as the "feel-good" neurotransmitter, plays a crucial role in regulating mood and promoting a sense of happiness and calm. Surprisingly, approximately 90% of the body's serotonin is produced in the gut, a revelation that underscores the gut's significant influence on mental health. This discovery reshaped my understanding of emotional regulation. When your gut is healthy and thriving, serotonin production is optimized, leading to improved mood and reduced anxiety levels. This connection between gut health and mental well-being is not merely anecdotal; it is grounded in scientific research (5) that continues to uncover the intricate relationship between these two realms.

The research revealed that individuals with a balanced and diverse gut microbiome experienced lower levels of anxiety and depression. It was a powerful reminder that nurturing your gut health could be a natural and effective way to support emotional resilience. This realization prompted me to delve deeper into the mechanisms at play. The gut-brain axis, a bidirectional communication network, allows signals to travel between the gut and the brain, influencing mood and cognitive function. Through this axis, the gut microbiome can produce neuroactive compounds that affect the brain's chemistry.

Understanding the gut's role in serotonin production is just the beginning of unraveling the complex relationship between gut health and mental wellness. The gut microbiome's ability to synthesize other neurotransmitters, such as dopamine, adds another layer to this intricate connection. Dopamine, known for its role in motivation and the pleasure-reward system, is also influenced by the gut. When the gut is in balance, dopamine levels are optimized, leading to increased motivation and a greater sense of satisfaction in daily activities.

As I explored further, I encountered stories from individuals who had experienced transformative changes in their mental health by prioritizing gut health. One account that stood out was of a young woman who struggled with chronic anxiety for years. Despite trying numerous therapies and medications, she found little relief until she began focusing on her gut health. By incorporating fermented foods, probiotics, and mindful eating practices into her daily routine, she noticed a gradual but significant improvement in her anxiety levels. Her story resonated deeply with me, underscoring the power of food and lifestyle choices in shaping our mental wellness.

The emerging field of psychobiotics, probiotics that specifically target mental health benefits, offers promising avenues for enhancing mental well-being through gut health. Clinical trials (9) have demonstrated the potential of certain probiotic strains, such as Bifidobacterium longum and Lactobacillus helveticus, in alleviating symptoms of anxiety and depression. These findings highlight the therapeutic potential of targeting the gut to support emotional resilience. While more research is needed to refine our understanding of the mechanisms at play, these studies offer hope for those seeking natural solutions to mental health challenges.

Reflecting on these insights, I am reminded of the profound agency we hold in shaping our mental health through the choices we make every day. By nurturing your gut health, you can lay the foundation for emotional balance and resilience. Simple practices, such as incorporating probiotic-rich foods into your diet, reducing processed foods, mindful food combining, and managing stress, can have a lasting impact on your mental well-being. This holistic approach empowers you to take charge of your mental health and fosters a sense of empowerment and hope.

Through my exploration of gut health and mental wellness, I have come to appreciate the profound interconnectedness of our body's systems. The gut's role as a "second brain" is not just a metaphor; it is a reality supported by scientific research and lived experiences. By prioritizing gut health, you can cultivate a foundation of emotional resilience, paving the way for a happier, healthier life.

How Gut Health Influences Immunity

Go back to that picture of the gut as a bustling metropolis, its inhabitants working tirelessly to keep the city thriving. Within this intricate system lies a powerhouse of the immune system, the gut-associated lymphoid tissue (GALT). This extensive network of immune cells forms the first line of defense against invading pathogens. The interactions between these immune cells and gut bacteria are critical. Beneficial bacteria help modulate the immune response, ensuring it is neither too weak nor excessively aggressive. This delicate balance is crucial in maintaining homeostasis, preventing inflammation that could lead to chronic conditions.

The relationship between gut microbiota and immune cells is a dance of communication and cooperation. Gut bacteria play a pivotal role in the activation and regulation of immune cells such as B cells and T cells. These cells are essential for identifying and neutralizing harmful invaders. B cells produce antibodies, while T cells directly attack infected cells.

Gut bacteria also produce metabolites, molecules that have anti-inflammatory properties, further aiding in the regulation of immune responses. This symbiotic relationship ensures that the immune system functions optimally, protecting against infections and diseases. The gut is not just a digestive organ; it is a critical player in your body's immune defense.

A balanced gut microbiome is a powerful ally in reducing systemic inflammation, a silent culprit linked to numerous diseases.

- Chronic inflammation is a ticking time bomb, quietly increasing the risk of potentially life-threatening conditions, including heart disease, diabetes, and even cancer. Fortunately, certain gut bacteria can help combat this inflammation. They produce short-chain fatty acids (SCFAs), which are known for their anti-inflammatory effects. These SCFAs promote a healthy gut lining and prevent the immune system from overreacting. By maintaining a balanced microbiome, you can reduce systemic inflammation and lower your risk of developing chronic diseases.

- Allergies have been linked to imbalances in the gut microbiota. A disrupted microbiome can lead to an overactive immune response, triggering allergic reactions. Similarly, autoimmune diseases such as celiac disease are closely tied to gut health. In celiac disease, gluten triggers an immune response that damages the gut lining.

In the vibrant landscape of your gut, the immune system operates with precision and purpose. Gut health influences immunity, inflammation, and disease resistance. By nurturing your gut, you are not only supporting digestion but also fortifying your body's defenses.

The Role of Gut Flora in Metabolism

Imagine your gut as a bustling marketplace, where goods are exchanged, consumed, and transformed into energy. This vibrant community is the home of your gut flora, a collection of microbes that play an intricate role in your metabolic health. These microorganisms are not mere bystanders; they actively participate in the complex process of energy extraction and storage. Short-chain fatty acids (SCFAs), produced by gut bacteria during the fermentation of dietary fibers, are not just byproducts; they are vital for regulating metabolism. They act as signaling molecules, influencing energy balance and the storage of fat. Through their action, SCFAs can enhance insulin sensitivity and promote a healthy weight.

The influence of gut bacteria extends beyond energy balance. They are pivotal in the absorption of nutrients, including essential vitamins and fats. The gut acts as a processing plant, where the fermentation of food leads to the release of nutrients in their absorbable forms. Vitamin D and calcium, for example, require a conducive gut environment for optimal absorption. When your gut flora is thriving, it creates the right conditions for these nutrients to be absorbed efficiently. This symbiotic relationship ensures that your body receives the nourishment it needs.

Gut bacteria also play a role in fat metabolism, breaking down dietary fats into components that can be used for energy or stored for later. This nutrient assimilation is vital for maintaining health and vitality.

But what happens when this balance is disrupted?

Long-term imbalance can result in metabolic disorders such as obesity and type 2 diabetes, conditions closely linked to imbalances in the gut microbiome. Research has shown that individuals with these conditions often exhibit distinct gut flora profiles, marked by reduced diversity and the prevalence of certain bacterial strains that promote energy harvest and fat storage. This shift in microbial composition can lead to insulin resistance, a hallmark of type 2 diabetes.

The presence of specific gut bacteria can influence how the body handles glucose, impacting blood sugar levels and metabolic health. Understanding this connection opens new avenues for addressing metabolic disorders, highlighting the importance of gut health in managing these conditions.

In a study (10) involving individuals who participated in a weight loss program, those who experienced significant changes in their gut microbiome composition also saw improvements in insulin sensitivity and weight reduction. This research underscores the potential of targeting gut health as a strategy for enhancing metabolic outcomes.

Another study (11) focused on individuals with type 2 diabetes, revealing that specific probiotic interventions led to improvements in glucose metabolism and insulin sensitivity. These findings illustrate the transformative power of a balanced gut microbiome in addressing metabolic challenges. They offer a beacon of hope for those seeking to improve their metabolic health through natural, gut-centered approaches.

By nurturing your gut flora, you create an environment conducive to metabolic balance. This involves consuming a diverse diet rich in fibers, prebiotics, and probiotics, which support the growth of beneficial bacteria. It also means adopting lifestyle practices that promote gut health, such as regular exercise and stress management. These practices work in concert to enhance the diversity and functionality of your gut microbiome. The journey to metabolic balance is not a solitary endeavor; it is a collaborative effort between you and the hidden ecosystem within your gut. In this pursuit, the gut becomes a partner in achieving optimal health and well-being.

Gut Health and Hormonal Balance

The gut is a master regulator of hormones, influencing various bodily functions in ways you might not expect. Picture your gut as a conductor, directing an orchestra of hormones to maintain balance and harmony within your body. Among the many players, estrogen and thyroid hormones are significantly influenced by the gut microbiome. Gut bacteria participate in the metabolism of estrogen, a hormone crucial for reproductive health and other bodily functions. They help in converting estrogen into its active forms, a process essential for maintaining hormonal balance. An imbalance in gut flora can lead to improper estrogen metabolism, potentially contributing to conditions like estrogen dominance, which is linked to issues such as weight gain and mood swings. Similarly, the gut's influence extends to thyroid function, where gut bacteria can impact the conversion of thyroid hormones into their active states, affecting metabolic rate and energy levels.

Stress hormones, particularly cortisol, are another area where gut health plays a pivotal role. When the gut is out of balance, a condition known as dysbiosis, cortisol levels can spike, exacerbating the body's stress response. Elevated cortisol can lead to a host of issues, from increased anxiety to disrupted sleep patterns.

Cortisol prepares the body to respond to a perceived danger or stressful situation. This works well when the danger is real, but we live in a world where there are constant stresses, and we have no outlet for cortisol to be used. Chronic stress means the constant production of cortisol, causing more bodily stress. The more stress, the more the body produces cortisol.

The gut-brain connection, while complex, reveals that nurturing gut health can be a powerful tool in managing stress. By promoting a balanced microbiome, you can help regulate cortisol levels, reducing stress and its impact on your body. Practices such as mindful eating, incorporating fermented foods, and reducing sugar intake can support this balance, paving the way for a more resilient stress response.

Reproductive hormones are also intricately linked to gut health. For women, the gut microbiome can influence menstrual cycle regularity and overall reproductive health. A balanced gut can aid in the regulation of hormones like estrogen and progesterone, essential for a healthy menstrual cycle. Meanwhile, gut bacteria can impact testosterone levels in men, affecting everything from muscle mass to libido. Maintaining a healthy gut can support hormonal balance, enhancing reproductive health and vitality. The complex relationship between gut health and hormones underscores the importance of a holistic approach to wellness, one that considers the interconnectedness of our body's systems.

To support hormonal balance through gut health, consider adopting a fiber-rich diet. Foods high in fiber, such as fruits, vegetables, and whole grains, promote the growth of beneficial gut bacteria. These bacteria aid in the detoxification of hormones, ensuring they are processed efficiently and effectively. Additionally, reducing stress is crucial for maintaining hormonal equilibrium. Techniques such as yoga, meditation, and deep breathing exercises can help manage stress levels, supporting both mental and hormonal health. Embracing these lifestyle changes can create a nurturing environment for your gut, allowing you to take control of your hormonal health and overall well-being. (See Appendix II: Learning to Meditate)

Incorporating these practices into your daily routine can lead to profound changes in how you feel and function. As you focus on gut health, you're not just addressing a single aspect of wellness; you're fostering a foundation for hormonal harmony. By understanding the gut's influence on hormone regulation, you empower yourself to make informed choices that support your body's natural balance. This approach not only enhances your physical health but also contributes to emotional stability and resilience. The journey to hormonal balance begins with the gut, and the potential for transformation is within your reach.

How Gut Health Influences Weight Management

Imagine your body as a finely tuned machine, where every component works harmoniously to maintain balance and function. Your gut flora, the collective ecosystem of bacteria residing in your digestive tract, plays a pivotal role in this system. These microorganisms are not merely passive inhabitants; they actively participate in regulating metabolism. They influence how your body extracts and stores energy from the foods you consume. For instance, certain bacteria break down complex carbohydrates into short-chain fatty acids, which are then absorbed and used as energy. This process highlights the direct impact of gut bacteria on your body's energy balance, affecting weight gain and loss. Research has shown that individuals with lean body types tend to have a more diverse gut microbiome compared to those who are obese. This diversity supports efficient energy extraction and utilization, contributing to a healthy weight. By nurturing a balanced and diverse gut flora, you can create an environment that supports your metabolic health and promotes weight management.

The intricate dance of hunger and satiety is also influenced by your gut. Hormones like ghrelin and leptin, which regulate appetite, are impacted by gut signals. Ghrelin, known as the "hunger hormone," is released when your stomach is empty, signaling your brain that it's time to eat. Leptin, on the other hand, is produced by fat cells and sends signals to your brain to reduce appetite when you've had enough to eat. These hormones work in concert to maintain energy balance, and their regulation is closely tied to the state of your gut. A healthy gut microbiome can enhance the effectiveness of these signals, helping you maintain a balanced appetite and prevent overeating. Neurotransmitters produced in the gut also play a role in appetite control, influencing mood and cravings. By fostering a healthy gut environment, you can support the natural regulation of hunger and satiety, facilitating weight management.

The connection between gut health and metabolic disorders such as diabetes is a topic of growing interest. Gut bacteria are involved in modulating insulin sensitivity, a key factor in the development of type 2 diabetes. Insulin is a hormone that helps regulate blood sugar levels, and when your cells become resistant to its effects, blood sugar rises, leading to diabetes. A balanced microbiome can enhance insulin sensitivity, aiding in the prevention and management of this condition. Additionally, inflammation, often exacerbated by an imbalanced gut, is a significant contributor to metabolic syndrome—a cluster of conditions that increase the risk of heart disease, stroke, and type 2 diabetes. By maintaining a healthy gut, you can reduce inflammation, improving metabolic health and reducing the risk of these disorders.

To leverage gut health for sustainable weight management, consider incorporating fermented foods into your diet. Foods like yogurt, kefir, sauerkraut, and kimchi are rich in probiotics, which help maintain a healthy balance of gut bacteria. These foods can enhance the diversity of your microbiome, supporting metabolic health and aiding in weight management. It's also important to use antibiotics judiciously, as they can disrupt the balance of gut bacteria and hinder weight management efforts. When antibiotics are necessary, consider taking probiotics to help replenish beneficial bacteria. By adopting these strategies, you can support your gut health and create a foundation for healthy weight management.

As we conclude this chapter, the intricate relationship between your gut and your body becomes evident. From influencing weight management to hormone regulation, the gut plays a vital role in maintaining your overall health. By nurturing your gut health, you unlock the potential for improved well-being and vitality. The journey doesn't end here. As we move forward, we will continue to explore the profound impact of gut health on various aspects of life, guiding you toward a healthier and more balanced lifestyle.

CHAPTER 3
COMMON GUT ISSUES AND THEIR ROOTS

IBS and Beyond:
Common Digestive Disorders

Have you ever felt a discomfort that you couldn't quite pinpoint, like a symphony out of tune playing in your stomach? That's how I felt when I first encountered the perplexing reality of Irritable Bowel Syndrome (IBS). It crept into my life subtly, manifesting as a persistent abdominal pain that seemed to have a mind of its own. The bloating, the unpredictable bowel habits—it was as if my body had decided to play tricks on me, leaving me frustrated and searching for answers.

IBS is a common disorder that affects the large intestine, manifesting in symptoms such as abdominal pain, bloating, and altered bowel habits. According to the Rome IV criteria, (12) IBS is defined by recurrent abdominal pain associated with defecation, a change in stool frequency, or a change in stool form. These symptoms can be deeply disruptive, impacting daily life and leaving you feeling isolated and misunderstood.

IBS is not the only digestive disorder that can throw your life off balance. Conditions like Crohn's disease and ulcerative colitis are also prevalent, each with its own set of challenges. Crohn's disease is a chronic inflammatory condition that can affect any part of the gastrointestinal tract, from the mouth to the anus. It often presents with inflamed patches interspersed with healthy areas, making it unpredictable and difficult to manage.

Ulcerative colitis, on the other hand, is limited to the colon and rectum, causing continuous inflammation and ulcers in the innermost lining. Both conditions can lead to severe symptoms, including diarrhea, fatigue, and weight loss, significantly impacting quality of life.

Another common issue that many individuals face is Gastroesophageal Reflux Disease (GERD). This condition occurs when stomach acid frequently flows back into the tube connecting your mouth and stomach, causing chronic acid reflux and heartburn. It's a sensation many of us have experienced, that burning discomfort rising through the chest, often aggravated by certain foods or stress. GERD can be a persistent nuisance, leading to complications if not managed properly. Understanding these conditions, their symptoms, and their impact on daily life is the first step toward finding relief and reclaiming control over your health.

Lifestyle and dietary choices play a critical role in the onset and management of these digestive disorders. Foods like dairy, gluten, and fried items can act as triggers, exacerbating symptoms and making management more challenging. For those with IBS, identifying and avoiding these trigger foods can be a game-changer. Stress is another significant factor, often overlooked in its ability to worsen digestive symptoms. The gut-brain connection means that emotional distress can manifest physically, leading to flare-ups and heightened discomfort. Recognizing these triggers allows you to take proactive steps in managing your condition, whether through dietary adjustments or stress-reduction techniques.

Management strategies for these disorders vary, but a holistic approach often yields the best results. For IBS, dietary adjustments such as a low-FODMAP diet (13) can be beneficial. This involves reducing intake of certain carbohydrates that are difficult to digest and can cause bloating and discomfort. Medications can also provide relief but should be considered alongside lifestyle changes for comprehensive management.

Probiotics, with their beneficial bacteria, can help restore balance in the gut, offering relief for some individuals. For conditions like Crohn's disease and ulcerative colitis, anti-inflammatory medications and immunosuppressants may be necessary, but dietary modifications and stress management remain crucial components of care.

With GERD, lifestyle changes such as avoiding late-night meals, reducing caffeine and alcohol intake, and elevating the head during sleep can make a significant difference. In severe cases, medications that reduce acid production might be required. However, the goal is always to find a sustainable way to manage symptoms and improve quality of life. Each of these disorders requires a personalized approach, as what works for one person might not work for another. Listening to your body and making informed choices are essential steps toward achieving digestive health and overall wellness.

Unpacking Food Intolerances and Allergies

As a chef, I have long wondered why food allergies and intolerances are becoming more common and why certain countries have significantly higher rates of specific food allergies. Imagine sitting down to a meal, only to be met with discomfort or even fear of a reaction. For many, this is a daily reality. Understanding the distinction between food allergies and intolerances is crucial in addressing these challenges.

Food allergies involve the immune system mistakenly identifying a food protein as harmful, triggering a defensive reaction that can be severe, even life-threatening. Symptoms can range from hives and swelling to anaphylaxis, requiring immediate medical attention. Peanut allergies are a prime example, where consumption can lead to rapid, dangerous reactions.

Food intolerances, however, don't involve the immune system. They arise when the digestive system struggles to process certain foods, leading to symptoms like gas, bloating, and diarrhea. Lactose intolerance, where the body lacks the enzyme lactase needed to digest lactose in dairy, is a common form of food intolerance. While discomforting, it doesn't pose the immediate threat that allergies do, allowing for more manageable solutions.

Food intolerances are surprisingly prevalent and can significantly impact daily life.

- **Lactose** intolerance affects a large portion of the global population, particularly those of East Asian, West African, and Mediterranean descent. Symptoms often include abdominal pain, bloating, and diarrhea after consuming dairy products. These symptoms can be disruptive, making social gatherings and meals challenging.

- Another common intolerance is to **gluten**, a protein found in wheat and other grains. It can cause digestive distress in those with celiac disease or non-celiac gluten sensitivity.

- Lastly, **histamine** intolerance, though less common, can lead to headaches, hives, and digestive issues.

Understanding these intolerances and their symptoms is a crucial first step in managing them effectively.

Accurate diagnosis of food intolerances and allergies is vital for effective management. For allergies, skin prick tests and blood tests can identify specific allergens by assessing the body's immune response. However, these tests aren't foolproof and sometimes require additional confirmation through food challenge tests under medical supervision.

Food intolerances, on the other hand, are often identified through elimination diets. This process involves removing potential trigger foods from the diet, then gradually reintroducing them to observe reactions. While effective, elimination diets require patience and careful monitoring. It's important to approach these methods with an understanding of their limitations and the guidance of a healthcare professional.

Once diagnosed, managing food intolerances involves making informed dietary adjustments.

- For those with lactose intolerance, lactose-free milk and dairy alternatives such as almond or oat milk can replace regular dairy products, with varying levels of nutrition.
- Gluten intolerances require a switch to gluten-free grains like quinoa, rice, and corn. These grains can be used in a variety of dishes, making the transition easier. It's essential to read labels carefully, as gluten can hide in unexpected places.
- For histamine intolerance, reducing intake of aged cheeses, fermented foods, and alcohol can alleviate symptoms.

These dietary changes, while initially daunting, can lead to a more comfortable and enjoyable eating experience.

Leaky Gut: Separating Fact from Fiction

Picture your gut lining as a brick wall, where tight junctions act as the mortar holding everything together. These tight junctions are crucial as they regulate what substances pass through your gut lining into the bloodstream. Now, imagine if this wall started to crumble, allowing particles that should stay within the gut to leak out into the bloodstream. This is the basic premise of 'leaky gut,' also known as increased intestinal permeability. The protein zonulin is thought to play a role in modulating these tight junctions, potentially increasing permeability. While this concept is intriguing, it's crucial to note its controversial status in scientific circles.

The link between a leaky gut and autoimmune diseases (14) has been proposed, suggesting that when the gut barrier is compromised, it allows larger molecules to enter the bloodstream. These molecules might trigger an immune response, potentially leading to autoimmune conditions. However, the scientific community remains divided. Some researchers argue that while the idea of a leaky gut is compelling, there is insufficient evidence to fully support it. Clinical trials yield mixed results, and many questions remain unanswered. This lack of consensus has led to debates about the validity of leaky gut as a diagnosis and its implications for health.

Symptoms attributed to leaky gut are varied and often vague, including fatigue, digestive distress, and brain fog. These symptoms are nonspecific and can overlap with many other conditions, making diagnosis challenging. Potential contributing factors to a leaky gut include chronic stress, an unbalanced diet, and excessive alcohol consumption. Stress, in particular, is known to affect gut permeability by altering the gut-brain axis. A diet high in processed foods and low in fiber can also compromise gut integrity by negatively impacting the gut microbiome. Understanding these factors is key to addressing symptoms and improving overall gut health.

Managing gut permeability requires a multifaceted approach, rooted in healthy lifestyle choices. A whole-foods diet rich in fruits, vegetables, and whole grains can support gut health by providing essential nutrients and fibers that strengthen the gut barrier. Incorporating fermented foods like yogurt and sauerkraut can also be beneficial, as they introduce beneficial bacteria that support gut integrity. Stress management is equally important; techniques such as meditation, deep breathing, and yoga can reduce stress levels and improve gut function. By focusing on these aspects, you can support your gut health without relying on unproven theories.

Understanding Inflammation in the Gut

Inflammation is often seen as an adversary, yet it is fundamentally a protective mechanism. When your body encounters a threat, such as an injury or infection, inflammation acts as a defense system, sending immune cells to the site to initiate healing. This acute inflammation is essential and short-lived, resolving as the threat diminishes. However, problems arise when inflammation becomes chronic. This occurs when the body continues to perceive a threat, leading to prolonged immune responses.

Chronic inflammation can silently simmer within the body, contributing to various health issues, including those affecting the gut. Within the gut, inflammation can disrupt the delicate balance of bacteria and weaken the gut lining, leading to conditions such as inflammatory bowel disease (IBD) and celiac disease. IBD, encompassing Crohn's disease and ulcerative colitis, is characterized by persistent inflammation of the digestive tract, where the immune system mistakenly attacks the gut lining, leading to symptoms like diarrhea, pain, and fatigue. In celiac disease, the immune response to gluten damages the small intestine's lining, impairing nutrient absorption.

Diet and lifestyle are powerful influencers of inflammation. Consuming a diet high in processed foods, sugars, and trans fats can fuel inflammation, while anti-inflammatory foods can help tame it. Foods rich in omega-3 fatty acids, like fatty fish, and those high in antioxidants, such as berries and leafy greens, can help reduce inflammation. Similarly, lifestyle choices like smoking and a sedentary lifestyle can exacerbate inflammation, while regular exercise and stress management can offer relief. Smoking introduces harmful chemicals that promote inflammation, while physical inactivity can lead to weight gain, further aggravating inflammatory processes in the body. By understanding these factors, you can make informed choices to manage inflammation effectively.

To reduce gut inflammation, consider incorporating anti-inflammatory foods into your diet, such as turmeric and ginger. These spices have been used for centuries for their healing properties and can easily be added to meals, such as curries and teas. Include more plants and fiber. Additionally, mind-body practices like yoga and meditation can significantly impact inflammation levels. These practices promote relaxation, reducing stress and the production of stress hormones like cortisol, which can contribute to inflammation. By integrating these dietary and lifestyle changes, you can support your body's natural ability to manage inflammation and improve overall gut health.

Interactive Element: Anti-Inflammatory Food Checklist

Consider keeping a checklist of anti-inflammatory foods you consume each week. Notice any changes in your symptoms or energy levels. This simple practice can help you stay mindful of your dietary choices and their impact on your gut health. Try adding new items to your list, exploring diverse foods that can support a balanced and inflammation-free gut environment.

Stress and Its Direct Impact on Digestion

In the quiet moments, when your mind races with thoughts of deadlines and responsibilities, you might not realize the significant impact stress has on your digestive system. The gut-brain-stress connection is a dynamic interplay that influences how your body processes and responds to the pressures of daily life. This connection, known as the gut-brain axis, allows your brain and gut to communicate intimately. When stress levels rise, your brain sends signals that can alter gut motility—the rate at which food moves through your digestive tract. This can lead to a range of digestive issues, from a sluggish digestive system that leaves you feeling bloated and uncomfortable, to an overactive one that results in frequent trips to the bathroom.

As mentioned in Chapter 2, stress also stimulates the production of cortisol, the body's primary stress hormone. While cortisol helps you manage acute stress effectively, chronic elevation of this hormone can wreak havoc on your gut health. High cortisol levels can disrupt the balance of gut bacteria, leading to dysbiosis, where harmful bacteria outnumber the beneficial ones. This imbalance can cause inflammation in the gut, exacerbating existing digestive disorders and creating a vicious cycle of stress and digestive distress. Cortisol also affects the production of digestive enzymes, making it harder for your body to break down food and absorb nutrients efficiently. This can lead to symptoms like indigestion, bloating, and nutrient deficiencies, further impacting your overall health and well-being.

The physiological effects of stress on digestion are profound. For individuals with conditions like IBS, stress can trigger flare-ups, intensifying symptoms such as abdominal pain, cramping, and diarrhea. The discomfort is not just physical; it often carries an emotional burden, creating anxiety about when and where symptoms might strike next.

Stress-related acid reflux is another common issue, where the pressure of stress causes stomach acid to flow back into the esophagus, leading to heartburn and discomfort. This can disrupt sleep and daily activities, compounding the stress you are already experiencing. Understanding how stress affects digestion is the first step in breaking this cycle and taking control of your gut health.

In the hustle and bustle of modern life, stressors are abundant and varied. Work-related stress is a significant factor, with tight deadlines, demanding bosses, and long hours taking a toll on your mental and physical health. The pressure to perform and achieve can lead to chronic stress, affecting not only your mind but also your body. Sleep deprivation, often a byproduct of stress, further compounds these effects.

Lack of sleep disrupts the body's natural rhythms, impairing digestion and contributing to weight gain and other health issues. The combination of stress and sleep deprivation creates a perfect storm, undermining your digestive health and overall well-being.

To support your digestive health amidst these challenges, adopting stress management techniques is crucial. Deep breathing exercises, particularly at bedtime, and progressive muscle relaxation can help calm the mind and reduce tension in the body. By focusing on your breath (not the mechanics of breathing) and releasing physical tension, you can create a sense of calm that benefits both your mind and your gut. Mindfulness-based stress reduction (MBSR) is another powerful tool, teaching you to live in the present moment and accept life's challenges with equanimity. This practice can help you become more aware of your body's signals, allowing you to address stress before it impacts your digestion. Simple practices like these empower you to take charge of your stress and its effects, paving the way for better digestive health and a more balanced life.

The Age-Related Digestive Decline

As we grow older, our bodies undergo a myriad of changes, and the digestive system is no exception. Aging can bring about a decline in the production of digestive enzymes, those essential proteins that help break down food into absorbable nutrients. You might notice that meals that once posed no problem now lead to discomfort or bloating. This is partly because the pancreas and other digestive organs gradually produce fewer enzymes, making it harder to digest and absorb nutrients efficiently. Additionally, the muscle contractions that move food through the digestive tract, known as peristalsis, tend to slow down with age. This reduction in gut motility can lead to prolonged transit times, meaning food takes longer to pass through your system. While this change is natural, it can result in uncomfortable symptoms like constipation and a feeling of fullness.

Common digestive issues, such as constipation, become more prevalent as we age, impacting our quality of life significantly. Constipation involves infrequent or difficult bowel movements, often leading to discomfort and a sense of sluggishness. With age, the frequency of bowel movements can decrease, and stool can become harder and more challenging to pass. This is not just an inconvenience; it can affect your daily activities and overall sense of well-being. Gastroesophageal reflux disease (GERD) is another condition that becomes more common with age. The relaxation of the lower esophageal sphincter—an important muscle that prevents stomach acid from flowing back into the esophagus—can lead to increased episodes of heartburn and acid reflux. These symptoms can disrupt sleep and lead to complications if not managed effectively.

Several factors contribute to age-related digestive changes and understanding these can help mitigate their effects. Medications commonly prescribed for conditions such as hypertension, arthritis, and depression can have side effects that impact digestion. Some medications can slow down gut motility, while others may alter the balance of gut bacteria, leading to digestive discomfort. It's essential to discuss any concerns with your healthcare provider, as they can offer guidance on managing these side effects. Reduced physical activity is another factor that can exacerbate digestive issues. Staying active helps stimulate gut motility, promoting regular bowel movements and preventing constipation. As we age, finding ways to incorporate gentle exercises like walking, swimming, or yoga into daily routines can be incredibly beneficial for maintaining digestive health.

To support healthy digestion as you age, making mindful dietary and lifestyle choices is key. Increasing your intake of fiber-rich foods, such as fruits, vegetables, whole grains, and legumes, can promote regular bowel movements and prevent constipation. Fiber adds bulk to stool, making it easier to pass and reducing the risk of digestive discomfort. Staying adequately hydrated is equally important, as water helps soften stool and supports the movement of food through the digestive tract.

Aim to drink plenty of fluids throughout the day and consider herbal teas or broths as additional sources of hydration. Probiotic supplements can also be a valuable tool for older adults, as they help maintain a healthy balance of gut bacteria. By introducing beneficial bacteria into your system, probiotics can improve digestive function and bolster your immune system, which naturally weakens with age.

As we navigate the complexities of aging, it's crucial to approach digestive health with a proactive mindset. Embracing a balanced diet, staying active, and addressing medication side effects can all contribute to a healthier, more comfortable digestive system. Remember, it's never too late to make positive changes that enhance your well-being. By focusing on these strategies, you'll not only support your digestive health but also improve your overall quality of life. With these insights in hand, we turn our attention to the next chapter, where we'll explore the role of nutrition in nurturing a healthy gut.

CHAPTER 4
GUT HEALTH ACROSS THE LIFESPAN

Nurturing Gut Health in Children: Building Immunity and Wellness

This chapter delves into the critical role of gut health in children, an area often overlooked yet profoundly impactful. As parents and caregivers, understanding and nurturing this aspect of health can set the stage for lifelong wellness.

Imagine watching a child's first tentative steps, their laughter echoing as they discover the world around them. Just as these early experiences shape their lives, so does the unseen world within them—their gut. From infancy, the gut is a vibrant ecosystem, bustling with activity as it lays the foundation for growth and development.

The significance of gut health in early childhood cannot be overstated. A balanced gut microbiome is essential for nutrient absorption, ensuring that children receive the vitamins and minerals crucial for their growth and development. This is particularly important for brain development, where nutrients like iron, zinc, and omega-3 fatty acids play pivotal roles. Studies have shown that a healthy gut is linked to better cognitive outcomes, affecting everything from attention span to memory and problem-solving abilities. The gut's influence extends beyond physical development, impacting behavior and emotional regulation. Children with a balanced gut microbiome often exhibit better social behaviors and fewer temperamental issues, highlighting the gut-brain connection even in early life.

To support a child's developing gut, dietary choices play a crucial role. Introducing a variety of fruits and vegetables not only provides essential nutrients but also prebiotic fibers that nourish the beneficial bacteria in the gut. These fibers, found in foods like bananas, apples, and carrots, act as food for the good bacteria, promoting their growth and activity. Including fermented foods like yogurt and kefir can introduce probiotics, live beneficial bacteria that help maintain a healthy balance in the gut. These foods are not only nutritious but also adaptable to a child's palate, making them an excellent addition to daily meals. Encouraging a diverse diet from a young age can help establish a robust gut microbiome, supporting overall health and immune function.

Note: Be sure the foods you buy for your baby does not contain added sugars, artificial ingredients, food dyes or synthetic fillers.

In today's fast-paced world, the convenience of processed foods is tempting, yet it comes at a cost to our children's gut health. Processed foods often contain artificial additives and preservatives that can lead to dysbiosis. This imbalance can compromise the gut's ability to function optimally, affecting digestion and immune response. Whenever possible, choose whole, organic foods that are free from these additives. These foods provide not only superior nutrition but also support a healthy gut environment, laying the groundwork for a lifetime of good health.

Fostering healthy eating habits in children requires creativity and involvement. Involve children in meal preparation, allowing them to participate in selecting ingredients and preparing dishes. This hands-on approach not only teaches them about nutrition but also encourages them to try new foods. Modeling healthy eating behaviors is equally important. Children learn by example, and when they see adults making nutritious choices, they are more likely to follow suit. Creating a positive, pressure-free environment around food can encourage children to develop a healthy relationship with what they eat, fostering habits that last a lifetime.

Interactive Element: Family Cooking Day

Choose a day each week for a family cooking session. Let children pick a recipe, gather ingredients, and help with preparation. Use this time to discuss the importance of each ingredient and its benefits for gut health. This practice not only educates but also creates cherished memories, reinforcing healthy habits in a fun and engaging way.

Managing Gut Issues During Adolescence

As a teenager, balancing school, social activities, and personal interests can feel like a juggling act. With peer pressure and the pressure to excel academically, stress becomes a constant companion for many adolescents. This stress doesn't just affect the mind; it also takes a toll on the digestive system. Stress-related digestive problems are not uncommon among teenagers, who often experience symptoms like stomachaches, bloating, or changes in appetite during exam periods or when deadlines loom. The gut-brain connection is real, and for teenagers, this means that stress can exacerbate existing gut issues, creating a cycle of discomfort and anxiety.

In addition to stress, adolescents today face a growing incidence of food intolerances. Whether it's lactose, gluten, or other dietary sensitivities, these intolerances can manifest as digestive distress, fatigue, or even skin issues. The challenge lies not only in identifying these intolerances but also in managing them within the context of a busy teenage life. Many adolescents find themselves navigating school cafeterias, sports events, and social gatherings, where food choices might be limited. This makes it essential for both teens and their parents to be aware of dietary triggers and to plan accordingly.

Balancing diet and lifestyle during these formative years is crucial for maintaining gut health. Despite hectic schedules, adolescents benefit from regular, balanced meals that provide the necessary nutrients to support growth and energy levels.

Encouraging the consumption of whole grains, lean proteins, and plenty of fruits and vegetables can make a significant difference. Hydration is another key aspect often overlooked. Busy days may lead to inadequate fluid intake, which can contribute to digestive issues and fatigue. Parents can play a supportive role by ensuring that water bottles are part of the daily routine, just like textbooks or sports gear.

Physical activity remains a cornerstone of adolescent health, offering benefits far beyond physical fitness. Regular exercise enhances digestion by promoting regular bowel movements and stimulating the gut's natural motility. Encouraging teenagers to engage in sports or active hobbies not only supports their physical health but also provides a healthy outlet for stress. Daily physical activity, whether it's a structured sport or a brisk walk, can help maintain a balanced gut microbiome, further supporting overall health. Adolescents who remain active tend to experience fewer digestive complaints, emphasizing the importance of movement in daily life.

Hormonal changes during puberty introduce another layer of complexity to adolescent gut health. Hormones fluctuate wildly during this time, impacting metabolism and digestion. These fluctuations can affect appetite, leading to overeating or undereating, both of which can upset the digestive system. Managing these changes requires patience and understanding. Adolescents should be encouraged to listen to their bodies, eat when they're hungry, and stop when they're full. It's also vital to address stress-induced digestive issues with strategies that promote relaxation, such as mindfulness or yoga. These practices can help calm the mind and, in turn, support a healthier digestive system.

Interactive Element: Stress-Reduction Techniques for Teens

Consider incorporating stress-reduction activities such as deep breathing exercises or a few minutes of daily meditation, which can make a significant impact. Encouraging teens to explore these practices can help them develop lifelong tools for managing stress and supporting their gut health.

Gut Health Strategies for Young Adults

The transition into young adulthood is often a whirlwind of change, with college, work, and newfound independence reshaping daily routines. Amidst these shifts, gut health can easily become a silent casualty. Irregular eating patterns emerge as a common challenge, with erratic schedules leading to skipped meals or late-night dining. The hustle of balancing classes or early work hours often results in breakfast becoming optional, while lunch is hastily grabbed between commitments. These patterns disrupt the body's natural rhythms, potentially leading to digestive discomfort and nutrient deficiencies. Fast food becomes an alluring option for its convenience, yet its high levels of unhealthy fats, sugars, and preservatives can wreak havoc on the gut microbiome. Over time, this reliance on processed foods can lead to imbalances, affecting not only digestion but also energy levels and mental clarity.

To navigate these challenges, young adults can benefit from strategic meal planning. Allocating time during the week to prepare meals can mitigate the tendency to resort to unhealthy options. Consider cooking in batches, creating nutritious meals that can be easily reheated. Emphasizing whole grains and lean proteins in your diet supports a balanced gut microbiome. Foods like brown rice, quinoa, chicken, and fish provide sustained energy and essential nutrients that keep your body functioning optimally. Incorporating plenty of fruits and vegetables ensures fiber intake, promoting digestive health and regularity. This approach not only supports gut health but also fosters a sense of routine amidst the chaos of young adulthood.

The pressures of young adulthood are not limited to schedules; stress is a pervasive factor that exerts a profound impact on gut health. Whether it's the demands of academic performance or the pressures of a new job, stress can lead to digestive issues like bloating, indigestion, and irregular bowel movements. Incorporating mindfulness practices into your daily routine can be a powerful tool in managing stress. Techniques such as meditation, deep breathing exercises, or yoga can help center the mind and calm the body, reducing the physiological impact of stress on the digestive system. Scheduling regular breaks throughout the day for relaxation, even if just for a few minutes, can help maintain a balance that supports both mental and physical well-being.

Social habits also significantly influence gut health during this stage of life. Young adults often find themselves in social situations where alcohol consumption is prevalent. While enjoying a drink with friends is a part of many social interactions, moderation is key to maintaining gut health. Excessive alcohol can irritate the gut lining and disrupt the balance of gut bacteria, leading to inflammation and discomfort. Being mindful of alcohol intake and opting for non-alcoholic alternatives can safeguard your digestive health while still allowing you to participate in social events.

Another habit to be mindful of is late-night eating, which can disrupt sleep and digestion. Consuming heavy meals close to bedtime can lead to acid reflux and poor sleep quality, further impacting your overall health. Aim to finish eating a few hours before going to bed, allowing your body time to digest properly. This practice supports not only your gut health but also your sleep hygiene, setting the stage for better rest and recovery.

Young adulthood is a time of exploration and growth and caring for your gut health ensures you have the energy and vitality to embrace this exciting phase of life. By adopting mindful eating practices, managing stress, and making informed lifestyle choices, you can maintain a healthy gut and support your overall well-being as you navigate this dynamic stage of life.

Adapting to Midlife Changes in Gut Function

As you enter midlife, your body begins to experience a series of changes that reflect the passage of time, and your digestive system is no exception. One of the most significant shifts is the decreased production of digestive enzymes. These enzymes, crucial for breaking down food into absorbable nutrients, become less abundant, making digestion a more laborious process. You might find that foods you previously enjoyed without issue now lead to discomfort or bloating. This change is a natural part of aging, yet it can be managed effectively with the right strategies. Alongside enzyme reduction, your metabolism—the rate at which your body converts food into energy—begins to slow down. This deceleration affects how efficiently you process nutrients and can lead to weight gain if dietary habits remain unchanged. The slower metabolism can also result in a feeling of fullness that lingers longer, which might seem beneficial but can actually signal a need for dietary adjustments to maintain energy levels and digestive comfort.

In response to these physiological shifts, adapting your diet becomes a crucial step in maintaining gut health during midlife. One of the most effective adjustments you can make is increasing your fiber intake. Fiber not only aids in regularity by promoting healthy bowel movements but also supports a thriving gut microbiome, which is essential for overall health. Incorporate a variety of fiber-rich foods such as whole grains, legumes, fruits, and vegetables into your meals.

These foods provide the bulk necessary for efficient digestion and help prevent constipation, a common challenge in midlife. Alongside fiber, incorporating healthy fats into your diet can offer anti-inflammatory benefits that soothe the digestive tract. Foods rich in omega-3 fatty acids, like salmon, walnuts, and flaxseeds, not only contribute to heart health but also enhance digestive function by reducing inflammation in the gut lining.

Lifestyle adjustments are equally vital in supporting digestive health as you age. Prioritizing regular mealtimes can help regulate your body's internal clock, promoting a smoother digestive process. Aim to eat at consistent intervals throughout the day, allowing your body to become accustomed to a routine that supports digestion. This regularity can prevent the overproduction of stomach acid and reduce the risk of acid reflux.

Don't overeat. Many people eat out of boredom or when their stressed. This can signal other issues that might be addressed by engaging in low-impact exercises such as walking or cycling. Being mindful of what you eat as well as how you eat can significantly benefit your digestive system. These activities stimulate intestinal contractions, promoting regular bowel movements and preventing constipation. Exercise also helps maintain a healthy weight, which can alleviate pressure on the abdomen and reduce the risk of developing digestive issues like GERD. By incorporating these gentle yet effective exercises into your routine, you support not only your digestive health but also your overall well-being.

Monitoring your gut health becomes increasingly important in midlife, as early detection of changes can prevent more severe issues down the line.

- Keep a journal to track your bowel habits: what time of day do you usually go, condition of stool, and note any digestive discomfort you experience. Notate changes in times and condition or appearance.

- Notate what you eat, how much you eat, how often you eat, and your frame of mind when you are eating. Are you stressed, bored, mindful?

This record can help you identify patterns or triggers that may be affecting your digestion. If you notice persistent issues or significant changes in your digestive health, don't hesitate to consult a healthcare professional. They can offer personalized advice and conduct necessary tests to ensure your gut is functioning optimally. Regular check-ups can also provide peace of mind, allowing you to address concerns before they escalate. Being proactive in managing your digestive health empowers you to navigate midlife with confidence, knowing you are taking steps to preserve your vitality and quality of life.

Supporting Digestive Health in Older Adults

As we age, our bodies undergo significant changes, and the digestive system is no exception. One of the primary challenges older adults faces is reduced gastric acid production. This decrease can hinder the stomach's ability to break down food efficiently, particularly proteins, leading to digestive discomfort and nutrient malabsorption. You might find that meals you once enjoyed now cause bloating or indigestion. Additionally, aging often brings increased sensitivity to certain foods, which can exacerbate these issues. Foods that were once easy to digest may now trigger discomfort, requiring adjustments in dietary choices to maintain digestive wellness.

To support gut health in older adults, focus on nutrient-dense foods that provide essential vitamins and minerals without overwhelming the digestive system. Incorporate lean proteins, colorful vegetables, and whole grains into your meals to ensure a balanced intake of nutrients.

As metabolism slows with age, energy needs decrease, making portion control crucial. Adjusting portion sizes can prevent overeating and reduce the risk of digestive distress. Smaller, more frequent meals can also aid digestion by reducing the burden on your gastrointestinal tract. This approach allows your body to absorb nutrients more efficiently and maintain energy levels throughout the day.

Hydration and fiber are key players in maintaining digestive health as you age. Regular fluid intake is essential for preventing dehydration, which can exacerbate constipation—a common complaint among older adults. Aim to drink water consistently throughout the day and consider herbal teas or soups as additional sources of hydration. Fiber-rich foods like beans, oats, and fruits provide bulk to stool, promoting regularity and preventing constipation. These foods support a healthy gut microbiome by feeding beneficial bacteria, enhancing overall digestive health. By emphasizing hydration and fiber, you can maintain a comfortable and efficient digestive process.

Establishing a consistent daily routine can greatly benefit your digestive health. Regular mealtimes help regulate your body's internal clock and can prevent digestive issues associated with irregular eating patterns. A routine that includes ample time for meals and relaxation can alleviate stress and promote better digestion. If constipation becomes a concern, consider natural laxatives like prunes, which can gently promote bowel movements. These strategies, combined with attentive dietary choices, can help you maintain digestive regularity and overall wellness in your later years.

Family-Friendly Gut Health Practices

In the rhythm of daily life, family often becomes the anchor that centers us. This bond extends beyond emotional connections, impacting our physical well-being, particularly gut health. By adopting a collective approach, families can weave healthy habits into the fabric of their everyday lives. Shared mealtimes are more than just an opportunity to connect; they are a chance to foster healthy eating habits. When families gather around the table, they model balanced eating for each other, creating an environment that naturally encourages healthier choices.

This practice not only strengthens familial bonds but also establishes a foundation for lifelong wellness habits. Moreover, engaging in collaborative grocery shopping can further deepen these habits. By involving everyone in selecting diverse, nutrient-rich foods, you can ensure that your pantry is stocked with ingredients that support gut health and makes everyone happy. This collaborative process empowers family members to make informed choices about what fuels their bodies, promoting a cycle of health-conscious decisions.

When it comes to crafting family meals, the goal is to create dishes that cater to all ages, making the table a welcoming space for everyone. Consider meals that are both balanced and gut-friendly, incorporating a variety of vegetables, lean proteins, and whole grains. For example, a colorful stir-fry with brown rice can offer an enticing mix of flavors and nutrients. Incorporating snacks that appeal to both children and adults, such as yogurt parfaits or whole-grain crackers with hummus, ensures that everyone enjoys delicious options without compromising on nutrition. These meals provide the necessary fiber and probiotics to support a healthy gut, while also appealing to different taste preferences within the family. By making mealtime a shared experience, you encourage everyone to appreciate the role of food in maintaining health.

Family activities also play a pivotal role in supporting gut health, providing opportunities for physical engagement that benefits everyone. Simple activities like family walks or hikes not only promote physical activity but also offer moments of connection with nature and each other. These outings can become cherished rituals that encourage movement, helping to stimulate digestion and support metabolic health. Gardening is another excellent way to engage the family while providing a source of fresh produce. Planting and tending to a garden foster a sense of responsibility and appreciation for where food comes from. This hands-on experience can teach children about the importance of nutrition and the benefits of consuming fresh, homegrown fruits and vegetables.

Education and awareness are key components in fostering a family culture that values gut health. Teaching children about the connection between food choices and well-being empowers them to make informed decisions as they grow. Encouraging curiosity about nutrition and health can be as simple as explaining why certain foods are beneficial or involving children in cooking. By cultivating an environment of learning and exploration, you instill a sense of ownership over their health. This knowledge equips them to make choices that support their overall well-being, laying the groundwork for a healthier future. As families embrace these practices, they create an environment where each member thrives, both individually and collectively.

By nurturing these habits, families can create a supportive environment that enhances everyone's well-being. As we move forward, we'll explore how these practices can be integrated into broader lifestyle changes that support holistic health.

CHAPTER 5
NUTRITION:
THE CORNERSTONE OF GUT HEALTH

Imagine a garden, brimming with vibrant colors, where each plant thrives in harmony, nourished by the healthy soil beneath with its plethora of vital organisms. Your gut health is much like this garden, where the soil represents the diverse community of bacteria that reside within you. As the gardener of your own body, the choices you make can either cultivate a flourishing ecosystem or disrupt its delicate balance. In this chapter, we explore the vital role of nutrition in nurturing this inner garden, focusing on the power of probiotics. These live microorganisms, found in certain foods and supplements, are the unsung heroes of gut health, fostering an environment where beneficial bacteria can thrive and support your overall well-being.

Probiotics 101: Choosing the Right Strains

Probiotics are living micro-organisms that have beneficial effects to their host. They can reduce constipation, help break down fat, and increase friendly bacteria in the gut, thereby boosting the immune system. But delving into the world of probiotics can feel like stepping into a bustling marketplace of choices. When it comes to probiotics, each strain offers unique benefits.

- **Lactobacillus acidophilus** stands out as a key player, known for its ability to aid in lactose digestion. For those who experience discomfort after consuming dairy, this strain can be a game-changer by breaking down lactose into more digestible components. This capability not only eases digestive discomfort but also encourages the consumption of calcium-rich foods essential for bone health.

- Bifidobacterium bifidum, another prominent strain, shines in its role of improving digestion. It helps maintain a balanced gut flora by inhibiting the growth of harmful bacteria, reducing the risk of infections, and promoting regular bowel movements.

- Saccharomyces boulardii, a beneficial yeast, offers protection against diarrhea, particularly that induced by antibiotics. It acts as a friendly soldier, reinforcing the gut's defenses and restoring balance during times of disruption. Exploring these strains reveals the diverse ways in which probiotics can support your digestive system, each offering a unique contribution to your gut health.

Selecting the best probiotic supplement is akin to choosing the right tool for a specific job. The efficacy of a probiotic is often measured by its colony-forming units (CFU) count, indicating the number of live microorganisms present. A higher CFU count generally suggests a more potent probiotic, capable of delivering a greater number of beneficial bacteria to your gut. However, it's essential to choose a supplement tailored to your specific health needs. For instance, if you struggle with lactose intolerance, a probiotic containing Lactobacillus acidophilus might be ideal. If you're recovering from antibiotic use, Saccharomyces boulardii could aid in restoring balance. Consulting with a healthcare professional can guide you in selecting a probiotic that aligns with your health goals, ensuring you receive the most benefit from these powerful allies.

While supplements offer a convenient way to introduce probiotics into your system, nature provides an array of delicious foods that are naturally rich in these beneficial bacteria. Yogurt and kefir are well-known for their probiotic content, offering a creamy and versatile base for smoothies, parfaits, or enjoyed on their own. For those following a plant-based diet, miso and tempeh are excellent sources of probiotics, adding depth and flavor to soups, stir-fries, and salads. These foods not only contribute to a diverse microbiome but also provide essential nutrients that support overall health. By incorporating these options into your diet, you harness the natural power of probiotics to maintain a healthy gut.

Incorporating probiotics into your daily routine can be as simple as it is enjoyable. Begin your day with a probiotic smoothie, blending yogurt with your favorite fruits for a refreshing and gut-friendly breakfast. Add a scoop of kefir to your cereal or overnight oats for an extra probiotic boost. At lunchtime, top your salad with a generous helping of sauerkraut, a fermented cabbage rich in probiotics, adding both flavor and gut benefits. And when preparing sandwiches or wraps, consider including a serving of kimchi, a Korean staple known for its spicy kick and probiotic content. These small, intentional choices can seamlessly integrate probiotics into your meals, supporting your digestive health with each bite.

If you're experiencing any of the following conditions, (15) it could be a sign that your gut flora is unbalanced or overgrown with harmful microbes.

- Food sensitivities
- Allergies
- Gas or bloating
- Weight gain

- Acne, eczema, rosacea
- Fatigue or weakness not due to exercise
- Mood swings
- Depression
- Autoimmune disorders
- Joint pain
- Anxiety
- Neurological impairment
- Difficulty sleeping
- Cognitive issues
- Persistent yeast infections
- Leaky gut syndrome or Chrohn's
- List of Probiotic FoodsKefir
- Yogurt
- Sauerkraut
- Kimchi
- Tempeh
- Some cheeses
- Kombucha
- Pickles

- Buttermilk

- Natto

- Miso

- Sourdough

Visual Element: Probiotic-Rich Food Chart

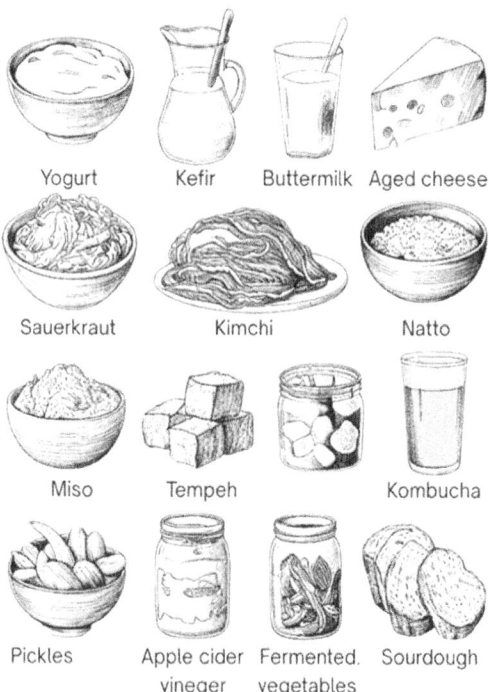

How many probiotic-rich foods from the list above can you incorporate into your diet? Display this chart in your kitchen as a daily reminder of the diverse and delicious options available to nurture your gut health. This visual tool can inspire you to explore new foods and experiment with probiotic combinations, making the journey to better gut health both creative and rewarding.

The Prebiotic Power: Fuel for Your Microbes

Imagine your gut as a bustling city, its inhabitants working tirelessly to keep the community thriving. Prebiotics are the unsung heroes in this metropolis, providing the necessary fuel for beneficial bacteria to flourish. Unlike probiotics, prebiotics aren't live bacteria, but rather fibers that nourish and promote the growth of healthy gut flora.

- Inulin, a type of prebiotic fiber, is found in various foods and plays a vital role in feeding these beneficial microbes. As it travels through the digestive system, inulin remains undigested until it reaches the colon. There, it serves as a feast for the good bacteria, stimulating their growth and activity.

- Fructooligosaccharides (FOS), works similarly by encouraging the proliferation of beneficial bacteria, which in turn helps maintain a balanced gut environment. By incorporating prebiotics into your diet, you create a nurturing environment for your gut microbiome, enhancing its ability to support overall health.

Everyday foods rich in prebiotics are abundant and accessible, making it easy to incorporate them into your diet. Garlic, onions, and leeks are not only culinary staples but also excellent sources of inulin, a fiber known for its digestive benefits. These foods add flavor to dishes while providing the nourishment your gut bacteria need to thrive. Bananas, often enjoyed as a quick snack or breakfast option, contain a unique combination of inulin and resistant starch, offering prebiotic effects that support digestive health. Asparagus, another prebiotic-rich vegetable, is versatile and can be prepared in various ways, from roasting to steaming. By including these foods in your meals, you naturally boost your prebiotic intake, fostering a healthy and diverse gut flora that can have far-reaching health benefits.

The relationship between prebiotics and probiotics is one of synergy, where each component enhances the other's benefits. When combined, they form what's known as synbiotics, a powerful team that works together to optimize gut health. Prebiotics provide the nourishment probiotics need to survive and thrive, allowing them to exert their beneficial effects more effectively. This partnership leads to enhanced diversity in gut flora, which is crucial for a robust immune system and efficient digestion. By incorporating both prebiotics and probiotics into your diet, you create a supportive environment where healthy bacteria can flourish, improving your gut health and overall well-being. This harmonious interaction highlights the importance of a balanced diet that includes both elements, ensuring your gut receives the comprehensive support it needs.

To make the most of prebiotics, consider integrating them into your daily meals with creative and flavorful recipes. A roasted garlic and leek soup, for example, combines two prebiotic powerhouses in a comforting dish that's both nourishing and delicious. By roasting the garlic and leeks, you enhance their natural sweetness, creating a rich and satisfying soup that supports your gut health. For a convenient breakfast or snack option, try banana and oat overnight oats. This simple recipe pairs prebiotic-rich bananas with oats, providing a hearty and gut-friendly meal that can be prepared in advance. By experimenting with these recipes, you can enjoy the benefits of prebiotics while savoring delicious, wholesome foods. These meal ideas not only support your gut but also add variety and excitement to your diet, making healthy eating an enjoyable and rewarding experience.

The following is a short list of prebiotic foods. There are many others.

- Chicory root – 47% inulin fiber; can e used as a coffee substitute

- Dandelion greens – 4 grams fiber per ½ cup; known for diuretic properties; has anti-inflammatory, antioxidant and cholesterol-lowering effects

- Garlic – 11% fiber from inulin; 6% fiber from fructo-oligosaccharides

- Onion – 10% inulin fiber, 6% FO.

- Leeks – 16% inulin fiber

- Asparagus - 2-3 grams fiber per ½ cup

- Bananas – 3-8 grams fiber per ½ cup; unripe bananas are high in resistant starch (prebiotic)

- Barley – 3-8 grams fiber per ½ cup; contains beta-glucan fiber; good source of selenium (helps thyroid and liver)

Interactive Element: Prebiotic Meal Planning Checklist

Consider creating a meal planning checklist that includes prebiotic-rich foods and recipes. Use this checklist to plan your meals for the week, ensuring you incorporate a variety of prebiotic sources into your diet. This tool can help you stay organized and motivated, making it easier to prioritize your gut health as part of your daily routine. The checklist will serve as a reminder of the diverse options available, encouraging you to explore new ingredients and flavors that support your well-being.

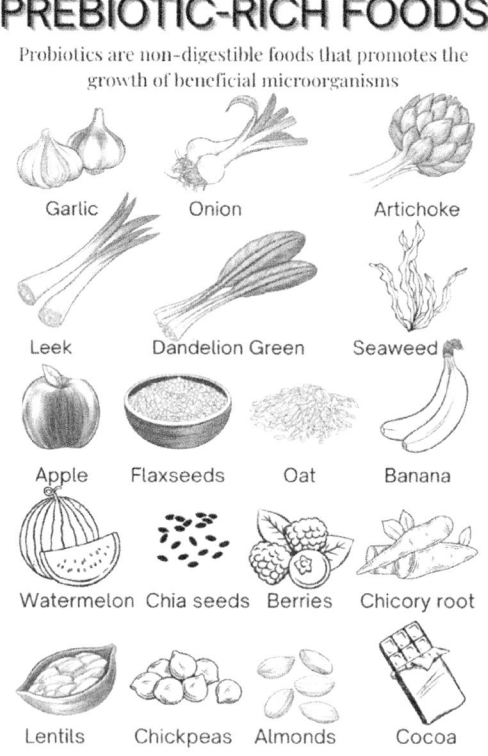

Designing a Gut-Friendly Plate

Imagine your kitchen table as a canvas, each meal an opportunity to paint a vibrant picture of health. Creating a gut-friendly plate is an art of balance, requiring a thoughtful mix of macronutrients—proteins, fats, and carbohydrates—that nourish your body and support your gut. Protein is the building block, essential for tissue repair and immune function. Lean meats, fish, beans, and tofu can provide this vital nutrient without burdening your digestive system. Healthy fats, found in avocados, nuts, and olive oil, are necessary for absorbing fat-soluble vitamins and providing sustained energy. Carbohydrates, particularly from whole grains, fruits, and vegetables, serve as your body's primary fuel source. The key is variety, not only in nutrients but also in colors. A colorful plate is not just visually appealing; it ensures a diverse intake of vitamins and minerals. By varying your colors, you naturally increase your consumption of different phytonutrients, which support overall health and well-being. Remember to keep proper food combining in mind.

Fiber is a cornerstone of gut health, playing a critical role in maintaining a balanced microbiome and promoting efficient digestion. Dietary fiber comes in two forms: soluble and insoluble, each with unique benefits.

- Soluble fiber, found in oats, beans, and legumes, dissolves in water to form a gel-like substance in the stomach. that binds to cholesterol before it enters the bloodstream. It helps regulate blood sugar levels while also feeding beneficial gut bacteria.

- Insoluble fiber is found in whole grains, nuts, and vegetables, and adds bulk to stool, aiding in regular bowel movements. It binds to cholesterol in the small intestine and pulls it out of the system.

Together, these fibers promote a healthy digestive tract, prevent constipation, and create an environment where beneficial bacteria can thrive. Consuming a mix of both types of fiber through a varied diet can enhance your digestive health, providing the foundation for a balanced gut ecosystem.

Water is another vital component of a gut-friendly diet, acting as the oil that keeps your digestive engine running smoothly. Our cells are comprised of 70-80% water. Without proper hydration, you cannot ensure that your digestive system will function efficiently

Water aids in the breakdown of food and the absorption of nutrients. It also helps maintain bowel regularity, preventing constipation and promoting a comfortable digestive experience. In addition to drinking water, you can increase your hydration through water-rich foods like cucumbers and watermelon. These foods not only provide hydration but also offer essential vitamins and minerals. By prioritizing water intake and incorporating hydrating foods into your meals, you support your digestive health and enhance your body's ability to process and utilize nutrients effectively.

Planning balanced meals throughout the week can seem daunting, but with a few strategic approaches, it can become a seamless part of your routine. Batch cooking and meal prep are powerful tools in maintaining a gut-friendly diet. Setting aside time at the beginning of the week to prepare large batches of grains, proteins, and vegetables ensures that you have nutritious options ready to go. This reduces the temptation to reach for processed or convenience foods that may disrupt your gut health. Incorporating seasonal produce into your meal planning not only adds variety but also ensures that you're consuming the freshest and most nutrient-dense options available. Seasonal foods are often more affordable and flavorful, enhancing your meals and encouraging you to experiment with new recipes and ingredients.

Interactive Element: Weekly Meal Planning Template

Consider using a meal planning template to organize your weekly meals. List out your breakfast, lunch, and dinner options, focusing on incorporating a variety of colors, macronutrients, and seasonal produce. This template can serve as a guide to ensure your meals are balanced and gut-friendly, making it easier to maintain a nutritious diet. You can rotate your menu during the month, keeping meal planning at a minimum once the initial work is done.

By planning ahead, you create a roadmap for healthy eating, empowering yourself to make choices that support your gut health and overall well-being.

Fermented Foods: Natural Probiotics

Picture yourself wandering through a bustling market, where the air is filled with the tangy scent of fermentation. This ancient process harnesses the power of microorganisms to transform simple ingredients into probiotic-rich wonders. At the heart of fermentation are Lactobacillus bacteria, which play a pivotal role in preserving and enhancing the nutrient content of foods. These industrious microbes convert sugars into lactic acid, creating an environment inhospitable to spoilage while simultaneously boosting the food's probiotic content. The result is not just preservation but a transformation that enriches the food with beneficial bacteria that can aid digestion and support a healthy gut.

Fermentation has been embraced by cultures worldwide, each with its unique contributions to this culinary art. From the spicy, vibrant kimchi of Korea, with its mix of cabbage, radishes, and chili paste, to the tangy sauerkraut of Germany, fermentation has been a cornerstone of traditional diets. East Asia offers us kombucha, a fermented tea celebrated for its refreshing effervescence and probiotic benefits. These foods carry the wisdom of generations, offering a taste of history and health in every bite.

Incorporating fermented foods into your diet can significantly enhance the diversity of your gut flora. A diverse microbiome is a marker of gut health, providing resilience against pathogens and supporting the immune system. Studies (16) have shown that regular consumption of fermented foods can improve microbial diversity, leading to better digestive health and overall well-being. Diversity indices, which measure the variety of microbial species in the gut, tend to be higher in individuals who frequently consume fermented foods. This improvement in gut flora diversity translates to enhanced digestion and nutrient absorption, as well as a strengthened immune system.

Fermented foods are not just a dietary addition; they are a cornerstone of a balanced gut ecosystem, supporting the body's natural defenses and contributing to overall vitality.

Incorporating fermented foods into your meals can be a delightful culinary adventure, offering both flavor and health benefits. Kombucha, with its fizzy and slightly tart profile, makes for a refreshing drink that can be enjoyed on its own or as a base for mocktails. Its probiotic content supports digestion, making it a perfect companion to meals. For a more substantial dish, consider kimchi fried rice. This vibrant Korean dish combines the bold flavors of kimchi with vegetables and rice, creating a satisfying meal that is both nourishing and gut friendly. The probiotics in kimchi enhance the dish's nutritional value, while the fermentation process adds depth and complexity to the flavors. Sauerkraut, with its tangy crunch, can be a versatile addition to sandwiches, salads, or as a simple side dish. Its probiotics can help balance your gut flora, supporting digestion and overall health. These creative uses of fermented foods not only provide variety to your meals but also contribute to a thriving and diverse gut microbiome.

Fermented foods are more than just a culinary delight; they are a testament to the power of nature in nurturing health. By embracing these age-old practices, you can enhance your meals and support your gut health in a delicious and meaningful way. Whether you're sipping on kombucha or savoring a bowl of kimchi fried rice, you're partaking in a tradition that has nourished countless generations. This connection to the past, coupled with the health benefits of fermentation, makes these foods a valuable addition to your diet, promoting a vibrant and resilient gut ecosystem.

The Anti-Inflammatory Diet: A Gut Health Ally

Picture a serene landscape bathed in calming colors, where every element exists in harmony. This is what an anti-inflammatory diet aims to achieve within your body, creating a state of balance that reduces the chaos of inflammation. At its core, this diet emphasizes whole, unprocessed foods, the kind that nourish without burdening your system with additives or chemicals. By reducing intake of inflammatory triggers like refined sugars and trans fats, you pave the way for your body to heal and thrive. This dietary approach is not just about avoiding certain foods; it's about cultivating a lifestyle that supports your body's natural defenses. It invites you to focus on what you can add to your plate, rather than what you must take away, fostering a sense of abundance and wellness. Whole foods, rich in nutrients and free from processing, form the foundation of this approach, supporting the body's ability to combat inflammation naturally.

Within this framework, specific foods emerge as powerful allies against inflammation.

- Omega-3-rich fish such as salmon and sardines are celebrated for their ability to reduce inflammation, thanks to their high content of beneficial fatty acids. These oils work to dampen inflammatory responses, supporting heart health and reducing the risk of chronic diseases.

- Vibrantly colored fruits and vegetables, like berries and leafy greens, offer an array of antioxidants, compounds that neutralize harmful free radicals and protect your cells from damage. The diverse pigments in these foods reflect a spectrum of nutrients that work together to bolster your health.

- Nuts and seeds, particularly flaxseeds and walnuts, provide essential fats and fiber, contributing to a well-rounded diet that supports both your gut and overall health. These foods are not just components of a meal; they are tools for building a resilient body, capable of withstanding the stresses of daily life.

The benefits of an anti-inflammatory diet extend far beyond individual symptoms, offering a holistic improvement in gut function. For those grappling with conditions like IBS, this diet can bring welcome relief, reducing symptoms such as bloating and discomfort. By supporting the gut barrier function, it helps maintain integrity and prevents the translocation of harmful substances into the bloodstream. This strengthens your body's first line of defense, minimizing the risk of further inflammation and promoting a sense of well-being.

An anti-inflammatory diet is not a quick fix; it's a sustainable approach that encourages long-term health improvements. Its emphasis on nutrient-rich foods supports a healthy microbiome, the community of microbes in your gut that plays a crucial role in digestion and immune function. By fostering a balanced gut environment, you create the conditions for improved health and vitality.

Incorporating these principles into your daily meals can be both practical and delicious. Imagine a warming bowl of turmeric-spiced lentil soup, where the golden hue of turmeric offers both color and anti-inflammatory benefits. Lentils, rich in fiber and protein, provide a hearty base, while turmeric's active compound, curcumin, adds a layer of healing potential. For a refreshing start to your day, a berry and spinach smoothie delivers a burst of antioxidants and nutrients, supporting your body's defenses from the inside out.

The sweetness of berries complements the mild flavor of spinach, creating a blend that's as nourishing as it is tasty. These recipes are more than just meals; they are acts of self-care, each bite a step toward a healthier, more balanced life. By embracing this approach, you not only support your gut health but also contribute to a broader sense of wellness that touches every aspect of your life.

Crafting Family-Friendly Gut Health Recipes

The family dinner table is more than a place to eat; it's a stage where relationships are nurtured and healthy habits are learned. Sharing meals as a family fosters a sense of belonging and connection, creating an environment where everyone feels supported. These moments of togetherness are opportunities to model healthy eating behaviors, showing children the value of a balanced diet and the joy of trying new foods. When children observe their parents making nutritious choices and enjoying a variety of foods, they are more likely to mimic these behaviors, setting the foundation for lifelong healthy eating habits. Incorporating gut-friendly foods into family meals not only supports individual health but also strengthens the family's collective well-being.

Creating meals that appeal to all ages requires creativity and a bit of strategy. Involving children in meal preparation can make a significant difference, transforming the kitchen into a space of exploration and learning. Let them wash vegetables, stir ingredients, or choose a new recipe to try. This hands-on experience encourages curiosity and investment in the meal, making children more likely to sample their creations. Balancing flavors and textures is another key to success. Pairing crunchy vegetables with creamy dips or mixing sweet and savory elements can create a dynamic plate that satisfies diverse palates. By considering the preferences and needs of each family member, you can craft meals that are both nutritious and enjoyable, making dinnertime a highlight of the day.

Kid-friendly recipes can be both nutritious and appealing, capturing the attention of even the pickiest eaters.

- **Homemade yogurt parfaits** with fresh fruit offer a delightful blend of flavors and textures, with layers of creamy yogurt, crunchy granola, and sweet berries. This dish is not only visually appealing but also rich in probiotics and antioxidants, supporting gut health while pleasing the palate.

- Another family favorite is **veggie-packed pasta** with tomato sauce. By incorporating a variety of colorful vegetables into the sauce, you create a nutrient-dense meal that children are more likely to enjoy. The familiar comfort of pasta serves as a welcoming base for the rich flavors of tomatoes, zucchini, and bell peppers.

These recipes demonstrate that healthy eating doesn't have to be complicated or boring; it can be a delicious adventure that the whole family enjoys.

Managing picky eaters can be a challenge, but with patience and creativity, you can expand their culinary horizons. Gradually introducing new ingredients is a gentle approach, allowing children to become familiar with different flavors and textures without feeling overwhelmed. Start by incorporating small amounts of a new vegetable into a favorite dish, gradually increasing the portion as your child becomes more comfortable. Creative presentation can also entice young eaters. Arrange food in fun shapes, use colorful plates, or create a theme for the meal. These small touches can make mealtime more exciting and encourage children to try foods they might otherwise avoid. By making meals visually appealing and engaging, you can transform eating into an enjoyable experience for the whole family.

This chapter has explored the powerful role nutrition plays in gut health, offering practical insights and ideas for creating a family-centered approach to healthy eating. As we gather around the table, we weave together the threads of connection, nourishment, and joy, fostering a culture of wellness that extends beyond the meal itself. In the next chapter, we will delve into personalized gut health protocols, exploring how tailored strategies can address individual needs and enhance overall well-being.

CHAPTER 6
PERSONALIZED
GUT HEALTH PROTOCOLS

The individuality within each of us extends to our gut health, where a personalized approach can make all the difference. One-size-fits-all solutions often fall short because they don't account for the unique composition of your microbiome, your genetics, or your lifestyle. Tailoring a gut health plan to your specific needs can be transformative, providing clarity and direction on your path to wellness. Understanding your body's specific requirements is the first step toward crafting a plan that truly supports your well-being.

Crafting a Personalized Gut Health Plan

Personalized nutrition is more than a dietary trend; it's a transformative approach that respects our individuality. Imagine two friends, both struggling with bloating. One finds relief by eliminating dairy, while the other benefits from reducing gluten. This variance isn't random; it's rooted in unique genetic makeups and lifestyle factors. If your family has a history of digestive issues, you may be predisposed to similar challenges. This knowledge can guide you in making proactive choices to mitigate potential problems. These differences underscore why a one-size-fits-all diet often falls short. By tailoring nutritional choices, we align eating habits with our body's distinct needs, paving the way for improved gut health and overall vitality.

The first step in creating a personalized gut health plan is conducting a thorough self-assessment. This involves taking a close look at your current health status, dietary habits, and lifestyle choices. This will require some work on your part, but it will be worth your time and effort.

Start by keeping a symptom tracking journal.

1. Record any digestive discomforts, such as bloating, indigestion, or irregular bowel movements.

2. Record what you ate before symptoms began.

3. Note the frequency and intensity of symptoms.

4. Look for patterns and match them against the foods you eat.

Complement your journal with a dietary and lifestyle questionnaire. Ask yourself questions like:

- How often do I consume processed foods?

- What is my stress level on a typical day? Do I eat when I'm stressed or because I'm stressed?

- Do I eat on the run or in my car?

- Are my meals balanced? Do I combine foods properly?

- Do I skip meals, eat when I'm not hungry, or eat quickly because I'm rushed?

- Do I become sleepy after eating?

By reflecting on these aspects, you gain a clearer understanding of the factors influencing your gut health. Tools to personalize nutrition have become increasingly accessible. Food sensitivity testing offers insights into which foods might be causing underlying issues. Although not definitive, these tests can guide dietary adjustments by highlighting potential irritants.

Dietary tracking apps serve as another valuable resource. By logging meals and symptoms, patterns emerge, revealing foods that may trigger discomfort or promote wellness. These tools empower individuals to take control of their gut health, offering clarity in a landscape often muddled by conflicting advice. With technology at our fingertips, personalizing nutrition becomes a manageable endeavor, not an overwhelming task.

With this foundation in place, you're ready to craft a personalized gut health plan. Begin by setting realistic, achievable goals. Whether it's reducing bloating, improving regularity, or enhancing energy levels, define what you hope to accomplish. Break these goals into smaller, manageable steps to keep yourself motivated and on track. Identify key areas for improvement, such as increasing fiber intake, incorporating probiotics, or managing stress more effectively. These focus areas will form the backbone of your personalized plan, guiding your daily choices and actions. Remember, the journey to optimal gut health is a dynamic process, requiring patience, flexibility, and self-compassion. Incorporating personalized nutrition into daily life requires a shift in perspective rather than drastic measures. It's about listening to your body's signals and respecting its unique needs. Start by observing how different foods affect you physically and emotionally. Use tools like food diaries or apps to track these reactions over time. Gradually, patterns will emerge, guiding you toward foods that truly nourish your body. In essence, personalized nutrition is a commitment to understanding oneself better. It's an ongoing process that evolves as you learn more about your body's preferences and responses.

Interactive Element: Self-Assessment Checklist

Create a personalized checklist to track your gut health journey. Include items like daily water intake, fiber-rich meals, and stress-reduction practices. Use it to monitor progress and adjust your plan as needed. This tool empowers you to take an active role in your health, fostering a sense of accountability and achievement. Embrace the individuality of your gut health journey, and let this personalized approach guide you towards a more balanced, vibrant life.

Tailoring Your Diet to Combat IBS

Living with IBS can feel like navigating a minefield of dietary triggers, where even a simple meal can cause discomfort. A key strategy for managing symptoms is the Low-FODMAP diet (Fermentable Oligosaccharides, Disaccharides, Monosaccharides, and Polyols), which reduces fermentable carbs that can trigger bloating and gas. While fiber is essential for digestion, choosing gentle sources like oats and chia seeds—and staying hydrated—helps maintain gut balance without irritation.

The Low-FODMAP approach involves eliminating trigger foods for 2–6 weeks, then systematically reintroducing them to identify personal sensitivities. The goal isn't permanent restriction but a tailored diet that minimizes discomfort while maintaining variety.

So, what can you eat on the Low-FODMAP diet? (17)

Category	High FODMAP Foods	Low FODMAP Foods
Grains	Wheat, Rye, Barley	Corn tortillas/chips, Grits, Gluten-free pastas/crackers/breads*, Oatmeal, Potato, Popcorn, Rice, Sourdough bread, Quinoa
Fruits	Apples/apple juice, Apricot, Blackberries, Cherries, Dates, Grapefruit, Mango, Pear, Watermelon	Banana (unripe), Grapes, Kiwifruit, Lemon, Lime, Mandarin orange, Orange, Papaya, Pineapple
Vegetables	Artichoke, Asparagus, Cauliflower, Garlic, Leeks, Mushrooms (button, portabella), Onion/shallots, Sugar snap peas	Bok choy, Broccoli, Carrots, Chives, Cucumber, Eggplant, Kale, Lettuce, Oyster mushrooms, Olives, Radish, Spinach, Tomato
Dairy / Plant-based	Coconut milk (carton), Frozen yogurt, Ice cream, Milk, Soft cheese, Soy milk, Yogurt	Almond milk*, Most cheeses, Coconut yogurt, Hemp milk*, Lactose-free ice cream/milk/yogurt*, Cottage cheese
Proteins	Most beans/legumes, Processed meats*	Edamame, Lentils, Canned/rinsed chickpeas, Beef, Chicken, Egg, Fish/Seafood, Pork, Turkey, Tempeh*, Firm tofu
Beverages	High fructose sodas/juices, Rum, Tea (Chamomile, Oolong, Fennel, Chai)	Wine (most), Beer, Spirits, Coffee, Sucrose-sweetened or diet soft drinks, Water, Other teas not listed above

Meal timing and portion control also play a role. Smaller, more frequent meals are easier on digestion, while avoiding late-night eating helps prevent flare-ups. IBS-friendly meals, like grilled chicken with quinoa and spinach or a Low-FODMAP smoothie with lactose-free yogurt and berries, show that gut-friendly eating can still be delicious. With mindful choices, you can nourish your body while keeping symptoms in check.

Supporting Gut Health in Aging Adults

As the years pass, your body undergoes changes that can affect every aspect of your health, including digestion. One of the primary challenges older adults face is decreased enzyme production. Enzymes are crucial for breaking down food into nutrients your body can absorb. Without enough enzymes, you might experience discomfort after meals, such as bloating or gas. This reduction often leads to altered gut motility, where the digestive tract's movement slows down. This slowdown can result in constipation, a common complaint among seniors. Recognizing these shifts is the first step in adapting your lifestyle to maintain digestive health as you age.

There are three types of enzymes: (18)

Food enzymes: These are found in all RAW foods. They come into the body through the raw food we eat or through whole food enzyme supplements. But food enzymes only work to digest the particular food it came from. Once food is cooked, all the enzymes are destroyed, so the body must produce enough enzymes to digest that food.

Digestive enzymes: These are secreted along the digestive tract and are mainly produced in the pancreas, but the liver, gallbladder, small intestine, stomach, and colon also produce enzymes. The five main digestive enzymes—proteases, peptidases, lipases, amylases, and nucleases—are produced in the body and aid in digesting the foods we eat and facilitating food absorption into the bloodstream. They turn food into energy the body can use for other biological processes and allow waste to be discarded. They are produced as the body needs them.

Metabolic enzymes: These are active protein chemicals found in all living cells, both plant and animal, and the 100 trillion cells in the human body all rely on the reactions of metabolic enzymes. There are about 1300 of these protein chemicals in the body and they can combine with coenzymes to create about 100,000 various other chemicals, all working to allow us to see, hear, feel, move, digest food, and think.

Metabolic enzymes occur at the cellular level, meaning they are produced by cells. Their main function is to transfer electrons from one molecule to another. They are produced as needed and catalyze and regulate breathing, heartbeat, and glucose, lipid and amino acid metabolism, to name a few. They are essential to every biochemical reaction in the body.

Taking digestive enzyme supplements can soothe digestive distress such as gas, bloating, and constipation, increase energy and absorption of nutrients, and promote regularity. If you want to take digestive enzyme supplements, be sure to use an enzyme product suitable for the type of foods you need to digest. For example:

- Lactase – Dairy
- Maltase – Starch
- Lipase – Fats (triglycerides)

- Sucrase - Sugars

- Amylase – Starches, complex carbohydrates

- Cellulase - Cellulose (vegetable fiber)

- Aminopeptide - Proteins

- Phytase – Phytates (beans, grains, nuts, seeds)

An enzyme deficiency will put a lot of strain on your body. What causes this deficiency?

- Not eating enough raw food. When we don't eat enough raw foods that contain enzymes (food enzymes) to aid in digestion, the body has to overwork producing more digestive enzymes to get the job done. As a result of this stressful demand on the body, the metabolic enzymes slow down, and every body system suffers.

- Processed foods. All industrially processed and packaged foods are devoid of enzymes.

- Cooking. Overcooking food kills most enzymes. If you're eating processed foods and then cooking or heating them, you're putting a huge strain on your body, which then has to provide the enzymes to digest the foods.

- Age and physical condition. The body produces fewer enzymes as we age. If your body is compromised in some other way, such as with illness or injury, the strain to produce enzymes is increased.

- Environmental factors. Pesticides, fungicides, herbicides, microwave cooking all contribute to destroy naturally occurring plant enzymes.

To address these challenges, consider incorporating more fiber-rich foods into your diet. Foods like whole grains, legumes, and vegetables can help maintain regular bowel movements and prevent constipation. Fiber acts like a gentle scrub brush for your digestive tract, keeping things moving smoothly. Additionally, staying active plays a significant role in promoting gut motility. Regular physical activity, even something as simple as a daily walk, encourages the natural contractions of your digestive system. This movement helps prevent the stagnation that can lead to discomfort and irregularity. Embracing these changes can significantly improve your digestive health and overall well-being.

Supplements can also be beneficial in supporting digestion for older adults. Probiotics designed specifically for seniors can help maintain a healthy balance of gut bacteria. These supplements introduce beneficial bacteria to your digestive system, aiding in nutrient absorption and reducing digestive discomfort. Digestive enzyme supplements are another option to consider. They can assist in breaking down food more efficiently, especially when natural enzyme production is low. Before starting any supplement, it's wise to consult with a healthcare professional to ensure they fit your unique health needs and conditions.

Eating well in later life presents its own set of challenges. Loss of appetite or dietary restrictions can make it difficult to get the nutrients you need. To enhance flavor without adding salt, experiment with herbs and spices like basil, rosemary, or turmeric. These can bring meals to life while supporting your health. Planning meals on a budget is another consideration. Batch cooking and freezing portions can make nutritious eating more manageable and affordable. Consider creating a weekly meal plan to minimize waste and ensure a balanced diet. By addressing these barriers, you can maintain a nutritious diet that supports your health and vitality.

Addressing Children's Gut Health Needs

Children's gut health is a cornerstone of their development. A robust microbiome doesn't just support digestion. It plays a critical role in building a resilient immune system. From a young age, the gut's ecosystem influences how the body responds to pathogens. It also regulates inflammation, offering protection against common childhood illnesses. The gut's impact extends to brain health, too. The gut-brain connection is vital for cognitive development. It influences mood, concentration, and even learning abilities. A healthy gut supports physical growth as well, ensuring nutrients are absorbed efficiently. This foundation is vital for a child's overall development and long-term health.

To nurture children's gut health, focus on a diet rich in diversity. Encourage the inclusion of various fruits and vegetables, each bringing unique fibers and nutrients. These foods feed beneficial bacteria, promoting a balanced microbiome. Limiting processed foods and sugars is equally important. These can disrupt gut balance, leading to issues like obesity and weakened immunity. Instead, opt for whole foods whenever possible. A colorful plate isn't just visually appealing. It represents a spectrum of nutrients that support a child's growing body. Building these habits early sets a foundation for lifelong health and wellness.

Allergies and picky eating are common challenges in children's diets. They can impact gut health if not managed thoughtfully. Allergies require careful dietary management. Identifying triggers and finding suitable alternatives is key. This ensures children receive the nutrients they need without discomfort. Picky eating can limit dietary variety, affecting microbiome diversity. Encourage adventurous eating by introducing new foods in fun and engaging ways. Make meals a family affair, where everyone tries something new together. Celebrate small victories, like a child choosing a new vegetable. These experiences can expand their palate and improve gut health.

Incorporating gut-friendly foods into a child's diet doesn't have to be a chore. Transform mealtimes into creative and enjoyable experiences. Try colorful, nutrient-dense smoothies. Blend berries, spinach, and a banana with a splash of almond milk. This creates a delicious drink packed with vitamins and prebiotics. For a treat, make homemade probiotic yogurt popsicles. Mix yogurt with pureed fruit, pour into molds, and freeze. These popsicles are fun and support digestive health. Engaging children in the preparation can spark curiosity and a love for healthy eating. They may even feel pride in creating their own snacks.

By focusing on gut health, you invest in a child's future. The habits formed now can impact their resilience to illness, cognitive abilities, and overall well-being. A diverse diet, mindful of allergies and preferences, supports a thriving microbiome. It creates an environment where children can grow and learn with vitality. As you guide them through these formative years, remember that each small step contributes to a healthier, happier future.

Managing Food Sensitivities with Precision

Imagine you're at a dinner with friends, and as you savor each bite, a nagging discomfort begins to creep in. This scenario underscores the importance of identifying and managing food sensitivities. These sensitivities can manifest in various forms, from mild bloating and gas to more severe reactions like migraines or joint pain. The long-term implications go beyond immediate discomfort. Chronic inflammation from untreated sensitivities can lead to more serious health issues, affecting both your physical well-being and emotional balance. Understanding this connection is crucial, as it empowers you to take control of your health.

Embarking on an elimination diet is a structured way to pinpoint food triggers. Begin by removing common culprits—such as gluten, dairy, and soy—from your diet for a set period, typically two to four weeks. During this time, monitor your body's reactions closely, noting any changes in how you feel. After this initial phase, carefully reintroduce foods one at a time, allowing several days between each new addition. This methodical approach helps you identify which foods your body tolerates well and which ones disturb your gut's harmony. It's a process of discovery, requiring patience and attention to detail. A food journal can be an invaluable tool in this journey, capturing the nuances of your body's responses.

Professional guidance is often essential in navigating food sensitivities. Dietitians and nutritionists bring expertise that can guide you through this complex process, ensuring nutritional adequacy as you adjust your diet. They can also help interpret the results of allergy tests, which may be recommended to pinpoint specific sensitivities. Allergy testing provides scientific backing, offering clarity and confidence in your dietary decisions. These professionals act as allies, supporting you in crafting a diet that not only avoids triggers but also nourishes your body and promotes overall wellness.

Living with food sensitivities requires a proactive approach, particularly in social settings. Reading food labels becomes second nature, as it's vital to ensure that hidden ingredients don't sabotage your efforts. Familiarize yourself with alternative names for common allergens and keep a list handy. When dining out or attending gatherings, communicate your dietary needs clearly and confidently. Most hosts and restaurants are accommodating when they're aware of your requirements. Carrying a small card that lists your sensitivities can be a discreet way to share this information. These strategies transform potential stressors into manageable situations, allowing you to enjoy social interactions without compromising your health.

Navigating food sensitivities might feel daunting at first, but with careful planning and support, it becomes a part of your lifestyle rather than a limitation. Embrace the opportunity to explore new foods and recipes, broadening your culinary horizons while keeping your gut health a priority. It's not just about eliminating foods; it's about crafting a diet that celebrates what makes you feel vibrant and alive. Each meal becomes a step towards better health, reinforcing the connection between what you eat and how you feel.

Troubleshooting Common Gut Health Challenges

Navigating the landscape of gut health can sometimes feel like walking through a maze, with progress hampered by unforeseen obstacles. One of the most common challenges is the frustrating plateau in progress where, despite your best efforts, symptoms persist. This can be disheartening, especially when you've been diligent in making dietary changes and lifestyle adjustments. It might feel like you're stuck in a loop, repeating the same steps without seeing the desired results. Another hurdle is maintaining consistency with these changes. Life's unpredictability often makes it difficult to adhere strictly to a new diet or routine, and the temptation to revert to old habits can be strong. This difficulty is compounded by the overwhelming amount of information and advice available, which can lead to confusion and uncertainty about which path to follow.

To overcome these obstacles, it's crucial to regularly reassess and adjust your dietary plans. What worked initially might need tweaking, as your body's needs can change over time. Consider seeking professional guidance if challenges persist despite your efforts. A healthcare professional or nutritionist can provide fresh insights and tailored advice, helping you navigate through the complexities of gut health.

They can offer a new perspective and introduce strategies you might not have considered, such as specific supplements or alternative therapies. This external support can be invaluable in breaking through the barriers that seem insurmountable on your own.

Patience and resilience are your steadfast companions on this path. Healing is seldom a linear process, and setbacks are a natural part of it. It's important to remember that progress, no matter how slow, is still progress. Setting achievable goals can help maintain motivation during these times. Celebrate small victories, like a day without discomfort or completing a week of consistent exercise. These milestones reinforce your commitment and provide tangible evidence of your efforts. Remind yourself of the long-term benefits and the improved quality of life that come with perseverance. This mindset will help you stay focused and optimistic, even when faced with challenges.

Preventing future gut health issues requires a proactive approach. Regular exercise is not only beneficial for your physical health but also plays a significant role in maintaining a healthy gut. It promotes regular bowel movements and reduces stress, which is often a trigger for digestive issues. Stress management is equally important; techniques such as mindfulness meditation or yoga can help keep stress levels in check. Consistent hydration supports digestion and prevents constipation, ensuring your gut functions smoothly. Balanced nutrition, rich in fiber and diverse in nutrients, provides the fuel your body needs to maintain a healthy microbiome. By integrating these practices into your daily routine, you create a supportive environment for your gut, reducing the likelihood of future problems. This holistic approach empowers you to take control of your gut health, fostering resilience against the challenges that may arise.

Building a Support System for Your Gut Health Journey

As you navigate your path to optimal gut health, it's crucial to recognize the power of a supportive network. Picture your journey not as a solitary endeavor but as a shared experience enriched by the presence of others. Friends and family can provide encouragement and hold you accountable, ensuring you stay committed to your goals. Their support can transform challenges into opportunities for growth. Imagine sharing a meal with loved ones, discussing the ups and downs of your gut health journey. These conversations can foster understanding and empathy, making your efforts feel less burdensome and more communal.

To build a network that bolsters your gut health aspirations, consider joining local or online communities dedicated to wellness. These groups can offer a wealth of shared experiences and insights, allowing you to learn from others facing similar challenges. Engaging with healthcare professionals, such as nutritionists or dietitians, can also provide valuable guidance tailored to your needs. Their expertise can help you navigate complex dietary adjustments, ensuring you make informed choices that support your health. Together, this network forms a safety net, catching you when you stumble and celebrating your victories, however small.

Social activities play a pivotal role in maintaining motivation and fostering a sense of community. Participating in group cooking classes or workshops can turn meal preparation into a fun, educational experience. These classes not only teach you how to create gut-friendly dishes but also connect you with others who share your health goals. Community fitness activities, like yoga or walking groups, offer a chance to engage in physical exercise while building relationships. These shared experiences create a sense of belonging, reminding you that you're part of something bigger than yourself.

Open communication about gut health is essential in building and maintaining these connections. Educating friends and family about the importance of gut health can inspire them to support your efforts and perhaps even join you on your wellness journey. Share your personal stories and experiences, highlighting the positive changes you've noticed and the challenges you've overcome. These narratives can motivate others to prioritize their own gut health, creating a ripple effect of wellness within your community. By fostering an open dialogue, you cultivate an environment where gut health is valued and prioritized.

As you reflect on the importance of a support system, remember that your journey is unique but not solitary. There is strength in numbers, and the collective wisdom and encouragement of your network can propel you forward. Together, you can create a culture of health and wellness that extends beyond individual goals, touching the lives of those around you. Embrace the connections you build, and let them guide you toward a healthier, more fulfilling life.

In the next chapter, we'll delve into the practical aspects of maintaining gut health, exploring how daily habits and routines can support your long-term wellness goals.

CHAPTER 7
THE FOUR-WEEK PROTOCOL: A ROADMAP TO GUT HEALTH EXPANDED

Week 1: Cleansing and Resetting Your Gut

Picture yourself standing by a calm, crystal-clear lake—the water still, pure, and inviting. That's exactly what this first week is all about: giving your gut a fresh start, a reset from the daily chaos of modern eating habits. This is your chance to gently detox, clearing out the processed foods and toxins that can slow you down. By doing this, you're creating space for better digestion, improved nutrient absorption, and a body that feels lighter and more energized.

So, what's on the "let's take a break" list?

- Added sugars, those sneaky ingredients hiding in processed foods that can feed bad gut bacteria and cause inflammation.

- Alcohol and caffeine, while they may be your go-to pick-me-ups, can be tough on your digestive system, so setting them aside for now gives your gut a chance to heal. Think of this phase as giving your body a well-deserved breather—it's not about restriction, but about making room for foods that truly nourish you.

- Water is your best friend—think of it as a gentle tide washing away toxins and keeping everything flowing smoothly. Aim for at least eight glasses a day, but more importantly, listen to what your body needs.

- Light movement, like yoga or a brisk walk, also helps by improving circulation and encouraging your body's natural detox pathways. And don't forget about rest.

- Sleep - This is one of the most powerful ways your body resets and repairs itself. Create a nighttime routine that helps you unwind—maybe a warm bath, a good book, or some gentle stretching to signal to your body that it's time to recharge. Quality rest makes all the difference in how you feel, helping you wake up refreshed and ready to take on each day. Create an environment that is conducive to sleeping.

- Stop using all electronic devices at least one hour before bedtime to eliminate the effects of blue light disruption.

- Keep the room dark.

- Don't work in bed. The bed is for sleeping, not for working. Don't return emails, catch up on social media, or get out that last document.

- Try to stick to the same sleeping and waking schedule every night. Lights out and screens off.

- If you wake up during the night, don't watch the clock. This will set off a cycle of thinking that makes it harder to fall back to sleep.

- Limit alcohol and caffeine, and don't eat heavily before bedtime.

By the end of this week, you'll likely feel the difference. More energy, less bloating, and a clearer mind—like wiping away fog from a windshield. As your body settles into this new rhythm, you'll start to notice an overall sense of balance and well-being. This is just the beginning of your journey, and already, you're giving your body the support it needs to thrive.

Reflection: Tracking Your Cleanse

As you step into this cleansing phase, consider keeping a journal to track your journey. Jot down shifts in energy, mood, and digestion, and reflect on how these changes make you feel. This simple practice deepens your connection with your body, offering both insight and motivation as you witness your progress unfold. Think of it as documenting your personal path to better health—one discovery at a time.

Envision this week as a refreshing rain after a dry spell, washing away what no longer serves you and creating space for renewal. By embracing this reset, you're not just supporting your gut; you're laying the foundation for lasting transformation. Approach this process with curiosity and openness, knowing that every choice brings you closer to a healthier, more vibrant you. This journey isn't about perfection but progress. Celebrate small wins, embrace the process with curiosity, and honor your body with nourishment, balance, and care.

Engaging Your Senses

As you progress through the week, engage more deeply with your senses, employing mindfulness not only at mealtimes but throughout your day. Consider how the process of detoxification feels within your body: each glass of water like a cleansing wave, each bite of food delivering nourishment. Engage with the sounds of your environment during walks or yoga sessions—the rustling leaves, the chirping birds—and let these sensory experiences ground you in the present moment, heightening the benefits of your detox journey.

Week 1 Meal Plan: Detoxifying with Purpose

So, what should you eat to support your gut and give it the cleanse it deserves?

- Start with a refreshing green smoothie—think kale, spirulina, and avocado blended into a creamy, nutrient-packed drink.

- Then, go for a detox salad loaded with beets, arugula, and walnuts, a perfect mix of fiber, liver-supporting compounds, and detox-friendly enzymes.

- Keep it simple yet nourishing with grilled lemon-herb chicken, steamed broccoli, and fluffy quinoa—balanced, satisfying, and full of gut-loving goodness.

- Spices and herbs are your secret weapons for both flavor and health benefits. A pinch of turmeric in your meals can help fight inflammation, while cinnamon adds a natural sweetness and supports blood sugar balance.

- And don't forget the power of small habits—starting your day with warm lemon water can do wonders for digestion and liver function.

- Add in gut-friendly cruciferous veggies like broccoli, cauliflower, and brussels sprouts, and you're giving your body everything it needs to detox naturally.

- To make this journey easier, a little meal prepping can go a long way. Chop your veggies ahead of time, marinate proteins for quick cooking, and batch-cook grains like quinoa or brown rice so they're ready when you need them. The more you prepare, the less time you'll spend stressing in the kitchen—and the easier it'll be to stay on track. Ready to give your gut some love? Let's do this!

7-Day Gut-Cleansing Meal Plan

Day 1

Breakfast: Green Detox Smoothie – Blend kale, spirulina, avocado, banana, almond milk, and lemon juice.

Lunch: Beet & Arugula Salad – Toss arugula, roasted beets, walnuts, and a lemon-olive oil dressing.

Dinner: Grilled Lemon Herb Chicken – Marinate chicken in lemon, olive oil, garlic, and herbs, then grill. Serve with steamed broccoli and quinoa.

Day 2

Breakfast: Cinnamon-Spiced Oatmeal – Cook oats with almond milk, top with walnuts and cinnamon.

Lunch: Quinoa & Roasted Veggie Bowl – Roasted Brussels sprouts, cauliflower, and beets over cooked quinoa, with a lemon-tahini dressing.

Dinner: Turmeric-Spiced Lentil Soup – Sauté onions, garlic, and turmeric, then simmer with lentils, carrots, and broth.

Day 3

Breakfast: Avocado Toast with Lemon – Whole-grain toast topped with mashed avocado, lemon juice, and walnuts.

Lunch: Broccoli & Chickpea Stir-Fry – Sauté broccoli, chickpeas, and garlic in olive oil, serve over quinoa.

Dinner: Herb-Roasted Salmon with Arugula Salad – Bake salmon with lemon and herbs; serve with arugula, beets, and walnuts.

Day 4

Breakfast: Spirulina Smoothie – Blend spirulina, banana, almond milk, cinnamon, and flaxseeds.

Lunch: Beet & Quinoa Bowl – Mix quinoa, roasted beets, arugula, and walnuts with lemon dressing.

Dinner: Cauliflower & Chickpea Curry – Simmer cauliflower, carrots and chickpeas in coconut milk with turmeric and spices.

Day 5

Breakfast: Turmeric Latte with Almond Milk – Warm almond milk with turmeric, cinnamon, and honey (if needed)

Lunch: Brussels Sprout & Walnut Salad – Shredded Brussels sprouts with walnuts, lemon juice, and olive oil.

Dinner: Passionfruit Garlic Shrimp with Broccoli & Quinoa – Sauté shrimp with garlic and gently toss with fresh passionfruit; serve with steamed broccoli and quinoa.

Day 6

Breakfast: Cinnamon-Spiced Chia Pudding – Soak chia seeds in oat milk, top with cinnamon and walnuts.

Lunch: Green Goddess Salad - Cooked shrimps, cucumber, celery and cherry tomatoes with homemade dressing

Dinner: Baked Herb Tofu with Steamed Greens – Marinate tofu in lemon, turmeric, and garlic, then bake; serve with arugula and steamed broccoli.

Day 7

Breakfast: Green Smoothie Bowl – Blend kale, spirulina, banana, and soy milk; top with walnuts.

Lunch: Falafel Salad with Tahini Dressing – Pan-fried falafel, tossed with chopped gem lettuce, sliced cucumber, radish, sun-dried tomato, coriander and tahini dressing.

Dinner: Grilled Chicken with Roasted Brussels Sprouts – Marinate chicken in lemon and herbs, grill; serve with roasted Brussels sprouts and cauliflower.

The Art of Mindful Eating

Think of this detox week as more than just a meal plan—it's an opportunity to slow down and truly enjoy your food. Set aside distractions, take a deep breath, and savor every bite. Notice the vibrant colors on your plate, the mix of textures, and the way each flavor comes together. Your meals aren't just fuel; they're nourishment for both your body and mind. Instead of aiming for perfection, focus on being intentional with each choice. Pay attention to how you feel—maybe lighter, more energized, or simply more in tune with your body's needs. Beyond digestion, this process can bring subtle yet powerful changes, like sharper mental clarity, steadier energy, and an overall sense of well-being. These little shifts are signs that your body is responding, guiding you toward what truly makes you feel your best.

Week 2: Reintroducing Nutrients with Purpose

You've given your gut the reset it needed—now it's time for the fun part! This next phase is all about reintroducing nutrient-rich foods in a way that nourishes and strengthens your system. Think of it like adding colors back to a blank canvas, one vibrant hue at a time, allowing your body to soak up all the goodness without feeling overwhelmed.

After cleansing, your digestive system is primed to absorb nutrients more efficiently, making this the perfect moment to fuel yourself with vitamins, minerals, and gut-loving foods that promote long-term balance and vitality.

So, what should be on your plate? Start with powerhouse nutrients that support gut health. Vitamin D plays a key role in immune function and helps beneficial bacteria thrive, while calcium works alongside it to support digestion, muscle function, and even neurotransmission. Then there's omega-3 fatty acids—found in salmon and other fatty fish—which help calm inflammation and keep your gut lining strong. These nutrients work together like a well-oiled machine, setting the stage for better digestion and overall well-being.

But remember, slow and steady wins the race. Reintroducing foods gradually gives your digestive system time to adjust without stress. Begin with small amounts of probiotic-rich fermented foods like yogurt or kimchi, helping to repopulate your gut with good bacteria. Then, ease into fiber-rich grains like quinoa or brown rice, which not only keep you energized but also act as prebiotics, feeding the healthy microbes in your gut. Taking it step by step allows your body to adapt comfortably, reducing any digestive discomfort and maximizing the benefits.

This phase is all about rebuilding and replenishing—nourishing your body with exactly what it needs to thrive. With each mindful addition to your plate, you're strengthening your gut, boosting your energy, and setting yourself up for long-term wellness. Enjoy the process, listen to your body, and embrace this exciting part of your journey!

Highlighting the Gut-Brain Connection

As you begin reintroducing nutrient rich foods, take a moment to appreciate the incredible connection between your gut and brain—often called the gut-brain axis. This powerful communication system means that what you eat doesn't just affect your digestion; it also plays a huge role in your mood, focus, and overall well-being. Ever notice how a nourishing meal can leave you feeling more energized and clear-headed? That's no coincidence!

Foods rich in probiotics and omega-3s—like creamy yogurt and flavorful salmon—help support mental health, reducing stress and boosting cognitive function. When your gut thrives, your mind follows suit.

This phase is also about tuning in and listening to your body's unique responses. Keeping a simple food journal can be a game-changer—it helps you track which foods make you feel amazing, and which might cause discomfort. Notice how you feel after meals: lighter, more energized, or maybe a bit sluggish? Even portion sizes matter! Sometimes, easing in with smaller amounts allows your gut to adjust more comfortably. Think of this as a conversation with your body—one where you're learning what truly nourishes and supports you.

Visual Element: Mindful Eating Journal

Consider creating a simple chart to track your meals and how your body responds, what I call "Mindful Eating Journal". Just a few columns—for the date, meal details, and any noticeable reactions—can provide valuable insights over time. It's all about learning which foods truly nourish you and which might need a second look. Think of it as a personal roadmap to better health, helping you fine-tune your diet in a way that feels right for you.

See the chart below as an example:

Date/Time	What did you eat?	What did you drink?	Physical activity	How much sleep?	What did you think?	How did you feel?

Importantly, be patient with yourself. This isn't a race—it's about building a way of eating that supports both your gut and overall well-being for the long haul. Approach each meal with curiosity, knowing that every small step you take is shaping a healthier, more balanced future. It's all about deepening your awareness of how what you eat influences how you feel. Each decision, each meal, is part of a bigger picture—your own personal wellness journey, where you are both the author and the main character.

The beauty of this phase lies in its simplicity: small, intentional changes that lead to lasting transformation. So, embrace this process, trust yourself, and let these insights guide you toward a future of vibrant health and vitality

Week 2 Meal Plan: Nutrient-Dense Choices

Think of your meals as a colorful canvas, with each dish adding a new layer of vitality. Start your day with oatmeal topped with berries and chia seeds, fueling your body with fiber and omega-3s. Then try a quinoa and chickpea salad—packed with plant-based protein and fiber. Together with wild salmon with roasted vegetables like sweet potatoes and Brussels sprouts, providing healthy fats and vitamins.

Variety is key! Swap in seasonal fruits, veggies, or different grains like farro to keep things fresh and exciting. Simple cooking methods like roasting and steaming help preserve nutrients, ensuring your meals are light and full of flavor. Boost your dishes with nutrient-rich seeds, like flax or pumpkin, and spices like turmeric for added health benefits. And flexibility is important—adjust meals based on your preferences or ingredient availability. This phase is how you enjoy your food while investing in your health and vitality for the future.

7 Day Nutrient-Rich Meal Plan for Gut

Day 1

Breakfast: Peanut Butter, Banana, Cinnamon Toast – Spread peanut butter on whole meal toast, top with sliced banana, and sprinkle over cinnamon powder.

Lunch: Quinoa & Chickpea Salad – Toss quinoa, chickpeas, arugula, and roasted beets with a lemon dressing.

Dinner: Grilled Lemon Herb Salmon – Marinate salmon in lemon, garlic, and herbs, then grill. Serve with roasted Brussels sprouts and sweet potatoes.

Day 2

Breakfast: Chia Pudding with Almond Butter – Mix chia seeds with almond milk and let sit overnight. Top with almond butter and blueberries.

Lunch: Bliss Papaya Salad – Mix fresh papaya slices with cooked green beans, sliced carrots, handful of roasted pumpkin seeds, cashew nuts and toss with fresh lime dressing.

Dinner: Baked Chicken & Brown Rice – Roast chicken with olive oil and herbs. Serve with steamed broccoli and brown rice.

Day 3

Breakfast: Creamy Blueberry Pecan Overnight Oatmeal – Combine oat milk, cover and refrigerate overnight. Add blueberries, pecan, and yoghurt when served.

Snack: Lunch: Roasted Veggie & Hummus Bowl – Serve quinoa with roasted carrots, zucchini, parsnips and chickpeas. Add a dollop of hummus.

Dinner: Tempeh Stir-fry – Sauté tempeh, bok choy, and ginger. Serve over cauliflower rice.

Day 4

Breakfast: Avocado Toast with Poached Egg – Top sourdough toast with mashed avocado, a poached egg, and microgreens.

Lunch: Vegetarian Black Bean & Lentil Burrito Bowl – Stir-fried sliced cabbage and onion; toss in cooked black beans, add chilli powder and lime juice. Serve over cooked lentil.

Dinner: Baked Cod & Asparagus – Season cod with lemon and herbs, then bake. Serve with roasted asparagus and quinoa.

Day 5

Breakfast: Whole-grain Banana Pancakes—Make the batter with whole-grain flour, egg, and almond milk and cook it over a hot pan. Serve with sliced banana and a dollop of yoghurt.

Lunch: Spinach & Chickpea Wrap – Toss spinach, chickpeas, chopped tomato and coriander in tahini dressing and wrap in a whole-grain tortilla.

Dinner: Garlic Shrimp Stir-fry – Sauté shrimp with garlic and herbs. Serve with brown rice and steamed broccoli, cauliflower and chopped parsley.

Day 6

Breakfast: Spirulina Smoothie Bowl – Blend spirulina, banana, almond butter, and chia seeds. Pour into a bowl and top with seeds.

Lunch: Grilled Tofu & Kale – Grill tofu, then serve with sautéed kale and roasted sweet potatoes.

Dinner: Poached Chicken & Melting Leeks – Slowly poach chicken breast and leeks log in chicken stock with turmeric, thyme, peppers. Serve over the mixture of yoghurt, grated garlic and chopped mint leaves.

Day 7

Breakfast: Green Scrambled Eggs & Whole-grain Toast – Scramble eggs with spinach, kale an green beans then serve on whole-grain toast.

Lunch: Wild Rice & Roasted Veggie Bowl – Combine wild rice with roasted vegetables and a lemon dressing.

Dinner: Miso Salmon & Barley– Marinate salmon in miso, then grill. Serve with stir-fried bok choy, brussel sprout and cooked barley.

Week 3: Balancing and Nuturing Your Microbiome

As we step into week three, the focus turns to the incredible ecosystem within you—your gut microbiome. Think of it as a flourishing garden, where balance and diversity create the healthiest environment. Beneficial bacteria like Lactobacillus and Bifidobacterium aid digestion, produce essential vitamins, and strengthen immunity. But when harmful bacteria take over, it can lead to digestive issues and weakened defenses. This week is about nurturing a microbiome that truly supports your well-being.

Start by incorporating prebiotics and probiotics into your meals.

- Prebiotics—found in foods like oats, asparagus, and garlic—feed the good bacteria, helping them thrive.

- Probiotics, found in fermented foods like yogurt, kefir, and sauerkraut, introduce beneficial bacteria, enhancing gut diversity. A mix of both creates a strong foundation for a balanced microbiome.

Beyond food, lifestyle choices play a key role.

- Chronic stress can disrupt your gut's balance, so prioritize relaxation through meditation, deep breathing, or time in nature.

- Sleep is just as vital—aim for 7–9 hours each night to keep your gut functioning at its best. Rest and restoration allow your microbiome to flourish, keeping digestion smooth and immunity strong.

- Get up and move, particularly if you have a sedentary job.

By making these small but impactful shifts, you're not just improving your gut—you're elevating your overall health. Let this week be about nourishing the invisible world within, creating balance that lasts far beyond these seven days.

Enhancing Microbial Diversity through Lifestyle

Gentle, consistent movement is a powerful way to support gut health. Activities like swimming, cycling, or even daily walks help improve circulation, enhance digestion, and promote microbial diversity. The key is to find exercises you enjoy—movement should feel energizing, not exhausting.

Spending time outdoors is another simple yet effective way to nurture your microbiome. Exposure to the natural world—soil, plants, fresh air—introduces beneficial microbes that enrich gut diversity. Whether it's gardening, hiking, or simply walking barefoot on grass, these small moments in nature can have a lasting impact on your gut health.

As you integrate these habits, take note of the subtle signs of a thriving microbiome. Regular digestion, stable energy levels, and even improved mood are all indicators that your gut is in balance. This is thanks to the gut-brain connection, where neurotransmitters like serotonin, produced in the gut, influence mental clarity and well-being. When your microbiome is flourishing, your whole body feels the difference—inside and out.

Interactive Element: Mindful Eating Exercise

This week, take a moment to practice mindful eating during at least one meal a day. Slow down, savor each bite, and tune into the textures, flavors, and sensations of your food. Consider how these nourishing ingredients support your gut health. Afterward, reflect on how you feel—physically and mentally. Small shifts in awareness can deepen your connection to your body's needs.

Balancing your microbiome is much like tending a garden—it requires patience, care, and consistency. Every nutritious meal, every mindful habit, and every moment of movement helps create an environment where beneficial bacteria can thrive. These daily choices don't just enhance digestion; they elevate your overall well-being.

As you continue this journey, stay curious. Explore new foods, pay attention to how they make you feel, and celebrate the progress you're making. Each step forward strengthens your gut, supports your mind, and builds a foundation for long-term health.

Week 3 Meal Plan: Cultivating Diversity

In week three, it's time to celebrate variety—both in flavor and nourishment. The main focus is on plant-based meals that bring richness and balance to your microbiome. It helps unlock a range of nutrients that strengthen your microbiome. Polyphenols in berries encourage beneficial gut bacteria, while fiber from legumes like lentils promotes regularity and supports overall digestive health. Each meal this week is an opportunity to nourish, restore, and energize your body from the inside out.

How about starting with a mixed berry parfait, layering crunchy granola and creamy yogurt? The berries, packed with polyphenols, act as antioxidants that help reduce inflammation and support gut health. Then, enjoy a comforting lentil and vegetable curry—hearty, fiber-rich, and filled with plant-based protein to fuel digestion and keep you satisfied.

Exploring New Culinary Horizons

Keep meals exciting by embracing global flavors. dishes like Korean kimchi stew, Indian yogurt lasi, or Japanese miso soup introduce beneficial bacteria while adding variety to your diet. Rotating ingredients—swapping quinoa for farro or spinach for kale—keeps your meals fresh and nutrient-rich.

Experimenting with international cuisines broadens both your palate and nutrition. Whether it's a hearty Italian minestrone or a spiced Indian dal, these dishes celebrate whole foods and bold flavors while supporting gut health. Seasonal produce adds another layer of nourishment—fresh, nutrient-dense, and bursting with flavor.

Cooking is both an art and an act of self-care. Play with spices like turmeric and cumin, which not only enhance taste but also offer anti-inflammatory benefits. As you explore new ingredients, stay mindful of how your body responds. Noticing how different foods make you feel deepens your connection to what truly nourishes you.

7-Day Gut-Healthy Meal Plan

Day 1

Breakfast: Chia Pudding with Almond Butter – Mix chia seeds with almond milk and let sit overnight. Top with almond butter and blueberries.

Snack: Greek Yogurt & Flaxseeds – A bowl of Greek yogurt with ground flaxseeds and a drizzle of honey.

Lunch: Vegan Coconut Curry and Pita. Bread – Saute onion, garlic, pepper, and zucchini, then add chickpeas and coconut cream. Simmer for 5 minutes. Serve with whole-grain pita bread.

Dinner: Baked Chicken & Root Vegetables – Roast chicken, carrots, asparagus, broccoli, parsnip with olive oil and herbs

Day 2

Breakfast: Berry Kefir Smoothie – Blend kefir, mixed berries, flaxseeds, and a drizzle of honey.

Lunch: Stuffed Sweet Potato with Hummus Dressing—Microwave sweet potato for 8 minutes, then split. Stuff with sauteed black beans, kale, and garlic. Top with hummus dressing.

Dinner: Grilled Salmon and Vegetable Skewers—Dice salmon, peppers, onion, and pumpkin into 2-3 cm cubes. Stick them on the skewers and grill until cooked.

Day 3

Breakfast: Turmeric Oatmeal with Walnuts – Cook oats with turmeric, cinnamon, and almond milk. Top with walnuts and fresh figs.

Lunch: Kimchi Brown Rice – Fry chopped garlic, kimchi, green beans and cooked brown rice. Serve with extra kimchi.

Dinner: Lentil & Spinach Soup – Simmer lentils, spinach, garlic, and tomatoes with vegetable broth. Serve with a side of fermented sourdough.

Day 4

Breakfast: Coconut Yogurt & Granola – Top coconut yogurt with homemade granola, pumpkin seeds, and pomegranate.

Lunch: Farro & Roasted Sweet Potato Salad – Toss roasted sweet potatoes, farro, arugula, and almonds with a lemon-olive oil dressing.

Dinner: Grilled Tempeh & Steamed Broccoli – Marinate tempeh in tamari, garlic, and ginger, then grill. Serve with steamed broccoli and quinoa.

Day 5

Breakfast: Capsicum Baked Eggs – Halve capsicums, remove seeds, crack in eggs, top with Mexican blend cheese and bake in the oven for 180C. Serve with sourdough slices.

Lunch: Wild Rice, Avocado & Seaweed Bowl – Mix wild rice with diced avocado, cucumbers, hemp seeds, and a lemon dressing. Top with seasoned seaweed flakes.

Dinner: One Pot Chicken & Vegetable Soup – Simmer chicken, ginger, turmeric, garlic, and carrots, tomato, brussel sprout, kidney beans in bone broth. Serve with brown rice.

Day 6

Breakfast: Mango-Kefir Smoothie – Blend kefir, mango, flaxseeds, and a pinch of cinnamon.

Lunch: Mediterranean Chickpea Salad – Mix chickpeas, cucumbers, tomatoes, olives, and feta with olive oil and lemon.

Dinner: Baked Cod with Roasted Cauliflower – Bake cod with garlic, lemon, and herbs. Serve with roasted cauliflower and quinoa.

Day 7

Breakfast: Scrambled Eggs with Spinach & Avocado – Scramble eggs with sautéed spinach. Serve with avocado slices.

Lunch: Miso Tofu & Soba Noodle Bowl—Marinate Tofu with miso, then fry. Combine soba noodles with miso broth, mushrooms, bok choy, and tofu. Sprinkle seasoned sesame on top.

Dinner: Stuffed Bell Peppers – Fill bell peppers with a mixture of quinoa, black beans, tomatoes, and cumin. Bake until tender.

Week 4: Strengthening Immunity and Longevity

As we enter the final week of this journey, our focus shifts to strengthening your body's defenses and embracing habits for long-term health. This week is about solidifying the foundation you've built and reinforcing your immunity to thrive for years to come. It's not just preventing colds—it's about empowering your body to resist various ailments and flourish.

Foods like garlic and ginger aren't only flavorful; they're powerful allies in boosting immunity. Garlic's allicin helps fend off infections, while ginger's anti-inflammatory properties support digestion and immune function. Citrus fruits, packed with vitamin C, also play a crucial role in maintaining skin health and promoting white blood cell production—your body's natural defenders. Including these in your meals can enhance your resilience.

Beyond food, lifestyle habits contribute to lasting wellness. Regular physical activity is key—it boosts circulation, helping immune cells flow through the body more efficiently. Whether it's a brisk walk, yoga, or a workout, movement invigorates both body and mind. Practicing gratitude and mindfulness is equally important. These habits reduce stress, a known immune suppressor, and foster a positive mindset, all of which promote longevity and overall well-being.

Building Resiliency Through Mindfulness

Resilience begins with daily mindfulness.

- Start your morning with a moment of stillness—whether through deep breathing, meditation, or quiet reflection. This simple habit helps lower stress and strengthens your immune system.
- Pair it with gratitude; recognizing small joys each day shifts your mindset, enhancing both mental and physical well-being. Sustainability is key. Lasting habits develop through small, consistent actions that seamlessly integrate into your lifestyle.
- Set realistic goals, check in on your progress, and adjust as needed. These mindful efforts reinforce the foundation you've built, ensuring your health remains a priority beyond this journey.

Picture starting your day with a warm cup of ginger tea, its soothing aroma signaling a fresh start. Imagine ending it with a gratitude journal, capturing moments of joy and progress. These aren't quick fixes—they're lifelong investments in your well-being. Take a moment to reflect on how far you've come. This journey has been about more than food; it's been about self-awareness, learning to listen to your body, and responding with nourishment, movement, rest, and reflection. Each step has contributed to a balanced, resilient approach to wellness. It's an ongoing practice of conscious choices.

As you move forward, carry this mindset with you. Every meal, every mindful breath, every act of self-care strengthens not just your immunity, but your overall capacity for health, happiness, and vitality.

Week 4 Meal Plan: Immunity-Boosting Recipes

This week, we focus on strengthening immunity through mindful nutrition. Think of each meal as a building block for resilience and longevity.

- Start your morning with a berry smoothie blended with flaxseeds—rich in antioxidants, vitamin C, and omega-3s to fight inflammation and support immune health. Pour it into a bowl, top with banana slices or almonds, and turn breakfast into a nourishing ritual.

- Then warm up with turmeric chicken soup, packed with curcumin's anti-inflammatory power and immune-boosting garlic and onions. Or have a simple yet nutrient-dense spinach and mushroom stir-fry, rich in folate, selenium, and essential vitamins.

Make meal prep effortless by batch-cooking soup or stir-fry, storing portions for busy days. Airtight containers help preserve freshness and nutrients, ensuring easy access to nourishing meals. As you savor each bite, see it as an act of self-care—fortifying your body from the inside out. Over time, you may notice more energy, a stronger immune system, and an overall sense of well-being. It's a commitment to long-term vitality and thriving health.

7-Day Gut Health Meal Plan

Day 1

Breakfast: Berry Flaxseed Smoothie – Blend mixed berries, flaxseeds, almond milk, and a touch of honey.

Lunch: Farro Salad with Arugula, Artichokes & Pistachios - Whisk lemon juice and oil in a salad bowl. Stir in farro, arugula, mint, basil, artichoke, and salt. Sprinkle with pistachios, pomegranate seeds, and goat cheese.

Dinner: Pan-seared Beef & Quinoa – Pan-seared beef with olive oil, garlic, and thyme. Add asparagus and Brussels sprouts to cook with. Serve with quinoa.

Day 2

Breakfast: Chia Pudding with Almond Butter – Mix chia seeds with almond milk and let sit overnight. Top with almond butter and blueberries.

Lunch: Creative Tuna Cesar Salad – For dressing, mix yoghurt, buttermilk, cheese, lemon garlic, and toss with radichio and gem lettuce, top with chunky pan-fried tuna.

Dinner: Turmeric Chicken Soup – Simmer chicken, garlic, onions, turmeric, carrots, and spinach in bone broth.

Day 3

Breakfast: Scrambled Eggs with Spinach & Avocado – Scramble eggs with sautéed spinach. Serve with avocado slices.

Lunch: Miso Soup with Tofu & Seaweed – Simmer miso paste in warm water, then add tofu, seaweed, and green onions.

Dinner: Stir-Fried Mushrooms & Brown Rice – Sauté mushrooms, garlic, and bok choy in sesame oil. Serve with brown rice.

Day 4

Breakfast: Oats with Cinnamon & Chopped Nuts – Cook oats with almond milk, cinnamon, and top with chopped walnuts and flaxseeds.

Lunch: Orzo Salad with Chickpeas & Artichoke Hearts – Marinade pickled artichoke with chopped chilli, garlic, parsley, olive oil. Toss in cooked chickpeas, ozro, spinach, cucumber cubes and crumble fetta.

Dinner: Baked Cod & Roasted Brussels Sprouts – Roast cod with olive oil, garlic, and lemon. Serve with roasted Brussels sprouts and quinoa.

Day 5

Breakfast: Coconut Yogurt with Granola & Berries – Top coconut yogurt with granola and fresh berries.

Snack: Celery Sticks with Almond Butter – Spread almond butter on celery sticks for a fiber-rich snack.

Lunch: Beef, Chickpea & Spinach Curry – Sauté beef slices, chickpeas, spinach, garlic, turmeric, masala spice in coconut milk. Serve with brown rice.

Dinner: Garlic Shrimp & Steamed Broccoli – Sauté shrimp with garlic, ginger, and olive oil. Serve with steamed broccoli and quinoa.

Day 6

Breakfast: Green Smoothie with Flaxseeds – Blend spinach, banana, flaxseeds, and almond milk.

Lunch: Roasted Beet & Goat Cheese Salad – Toss roasted beets, goat cheese, arugula, and walnuts with balsamic dressing.

Dinner: Sesame Kohlrabi & Prawn – For dressing, whisk vinegar, tamari, chile-garlic sauce, orange zest, grapeseed and sesame oil. Stir in kohlrabi, cabbage, cooked prawns, carrots and snow peas. Serve topped with almonds, sesame seeds and cilantro.

Day 7

Breakfast: Kefir with Mixed Nuts & Seeds – Pour kefir into a bowl and top with almonds, walnuts, and pumpkin seeds.

Lunch: Chicken Waldorf Salad – For dressing, mix yoghurt, buttermilk, cheese, lemon garlic. Mix diced cooked chicken breast, diced apples, celery, cherry tomato, roasted walnut and dressing.

Dinner: Mushroom & Spinach Stir-Fry – Sauté mushrooms, spinach, and garlic in sesame oil. Serve with brown rice.

The Role of Supplements: When and How to Use Them

Supplements can be powerful allies in your gut health journey, but they're not magic fixes. Think of them as tools that support your body—filling nutritional gaps, improving digestion, and strengthening your microbiome. When chosen wisely, they can enhance your efforts, but they should never replace a nutrient-rich, whole-food diet.

- Probiotics are one of the most well-known gut health supplements, helping restore balance to your microbiome after illness, antibiotics, or dietary imbalances.
- Digestive enzymes can also be beneficial, easing bloating and improving nutrient absorption, especially for those with food intolerances.
- Adaptogens are substances that help to restore balance in stressed areas of the body. Ashwagandha, holy basil, and reishi are good examples that may further support gut health by helping your body adapt to stress—a key factor in digestive well-being.

When choosing supplements, quality matters. Look for trusted brands that begin with whole food, with transparent ingredients and third-party testing, and consult a healthcare professional to ensure they align with your individual needs. More isn't always better—overuse can lead to imbalances, so start slow and pay attention to how your body responds.

Supplements should enhance, not overshadow, the foundation of good health: whole foods, movement, rest, and stress management. Think of them as one piece of a bigger picture—supporting your body's natural ability to heal, protect, and thrive. By making informed, mindful choices, you empower yourself to take control of your gut health and overall well-being.

Tracking Progress: Assessing Your Gut Health Journey

Tracking your progress is a plan and understanding what works for you. Think of it as a compass guiding your gut health journey, helping you make informed adjustments along the way. A simple food diary can reveal valuable patterns by linking what you eat to how you feel.

Digital tracking apps offer a convenient way to log meals and symptoms, making it easier to spot triggers and supportive foods. Beyond diet, consider noting stress levels, emotions, and sleep—since gut health is deeply connected to overall well-being, these insights can provide a more complete picture.

Progress isn't just the absence of discomfort; it's the presence of positive changes. Notice shifts in digestion, energy, and mood. If certain foods consistently cause discomfort, adjust accordingly. If something makes you feel great, lean into it. Long-term success comes from maintaining momentum. Once your initial protocol ends, set new health goals—experiment with new recipes, explore different movement practices, or deepen your gut health knowledge. Consistency is key. By embracing gut health as an ongoing journey rather than a fixed destination, you create a lifestyle that nurtures both your body and mind.

CHAPTER 8
LIFESTYLE AND THE GUT HEALTH CONNECTION

How Hydration Affects Digestion

Picture a serene river, its waters flowing steadily, nourishing the land it passes. Your body is much like this river, reliant on a constant flow of water to maintain balance and vitality. Water is not just a thirst quencher; it is the unsung hero of digestion. It helps break down food, making nutrients accessible and aiding their absorption into your bloodstream. Without sufficient hydration, digestion becomes sluggish, akin to a river that slows to a trickle, filled with debris and unable to sustain the life around it. This slowdown can lead to constipation, where waste moves like a tortoise through your intestines, causing discomfort and frustration.

Dehydrated, your digestive system struggles, its mucosal lining weakened, leaving it vulnerable to irritants and infections. The gut's protective barrier, essential for keeping harmful substances at bay, falters, increasing susceptibility to digestive issues. Ensuring adequate hydration is like tending to a garden; it requires consistent care and attention.

You might wonder how much water is enough. While there's no one-size-fits-all answer, a good rule of thumb is to pay attention to your body's signals. Drink consistently throughout the day, rather than waiting for thirst to strike. Incorporate hydrating foods, like cucumbers, tomatoes and watermelon, into your meals. These foods not only provide fluids but also offer vitamins and minerals that support overall health.

Staying hydrated doesn't have to be a chore. Simple strategies can help you make it a natural part of your routine. Consider carrying a water bottle with measurement markers, a tangible reminder of your daily intake goals. Set reminders on your phone to prompt you to drink at regular intervals. These small changes can have a profound impact on your gut health and overall well-being.

Interactive Element: Hydration Challenge

Set a daily goal for water intake. Some experts recommend starting with one ounce of water for every two pounds of body weight, adjusting for activity levels and any illness and medication. Use a journal to track your progress, noting any changes in energy levels or digestion. Reflect on the connection between your hydration habits and how you feel.

In the grand tapestry of wellness, hydration is a thread that weaves through every aspect of health. Our cells are 70% water, so it's not just about quenching thirst; it's about fostering an environment where your body and mind can do what they're intended to do and flourish. Embrace this simple yet powerful tool, and let it guide you toward a more vibrant, balanced life.

The Sleep-Digestion Connection

Think about the last time you tossed and turned all night, only to wake up feeling groggy and out of sorts. It's a sensation that's all too familiar for many, and its effects ripple far beyond fatigue. Poor sleep does more than sap your energy; it disrupts your digestive processes, altering the gut microbiome in ways that can lead to a cascade of health issues. Sleep deprivation has been shown to reduce the diversity of beneficial bacteria in your gut, tipping the balance in favor of harmful strains. This imbalance can contribute to inflammation, weaken your immune system, and leave you more susceptible to infections and digestive disorders like irritable bowel syndrome (IBS). It's a stark reminder that restful sleep is more than a luxury—it's a cornerstone of digestive health.

The body's internal clock, or circadian rhythm, orchestrates a delicate symphony of biological processes, digestion included. This rhythm regulates the release of hormones that influence hunger and satiety, such as ghrelin and leptin, aligning them with day and night cycles. When your circadian rhythms are disrupted, perhaps by irregular sleep patterns or late-night snacking, this hormonal harmony falters. You might find yourself craving unhealthy foods at odd hours or feeling hungry when you should be winding down. This misalignment can lead to poor food choices, exacerbating digestive issues.

Timing your meals to coincide with your body's natural rhythms can enhance digestive efficiency and nutrient absorption. Eating substantial meals earlier in the day, when your metabolism is more active, can support better digestion and contribute to a healthier gut microbiome.

Sleep disturbances like insomnia and sleep apnea are culprits that further complicate your digestive health. Insomnia often leads to increased stress and anxiety, both of which can exacerbate gastrointestinal discomfort. The lack of sleep can also heighten your sensitivity to pain, making symptoms of digestive disorders more pronounced. Sleep apnea, marked by interrupted breathing during sleep, has a direct link to acid reflux. The pauses in breathing can cause pressure changes in the esophagus, allowing stomach acid to flow back upward. This not only disrupts sleep but also exacerbates GERD symptoms, creating a vicious cycle. Addressing these sleep issues can bring relief to your digestive system and improve your overall quality of life.

Achieving restful sleep that supports digestion involves a few simple, yet effective strategies.

- Start by establishing a consistent sleep schedule, going to bed and waking up at the same time every day, even on weekends. This consistency reinforces your body's natural sleep-wake cycle, making it easier to fall and stay asleep.

- Create a calming bedtime routine to prepare your mind and body for rest. Consider activities like reading, gentle stretching, or meditation to signal to your body that it's time to wind down.

- Minimize caffeine and heavy meals before bedtime, as these can disrupt sleep and digestion. A light evening meal, eaten a few hours before bed, allows your digestive system to process food without strain, promoting a more restful night.

- Keep your bedroom dark by eliminating light coming from outside and turning off electronics.

- Incorporate the Amish Hour: stop using all electronics one hour before bedtime, including TV, phones, and computers.

Stress Management Techniques for Better Gut Health

Stress is an all-too-familiar companion in modern life, often lurking in the background as a silent saboteur of well-being. Its impact stretches far beyond the mind, reaching deep into the gut where it can wreak havoc on digestive health. Prolonged stress is known to alter gut permeability, a phenomenon where the once-tight junctions in the gut lining loosen, allowing unwelcome particles to pass through. This not only triggers inflammation but can also exacerbate conditions like irritable bowel syndrome (IBS), where stress is a well-documented trigger. The result is a vicious cycle: stress aggravates gut issues, which then increase stress, trapping you in a loop of discomfort and anxiety.

To break free, incorporating effective stress-reduction techniques into your routine is crucial.

- Progressive muscle relaxation, a practice that involves tensing and then slowly releasing each muscle group in the body, helps to calm the nervous system, reducing stress and its physical manifestations in the gut.

- Journaling is a powerful tool. By putting pen to paper, you can externalize your worries, gaining perspective and clarity. This simple act of reflection can be cathartic, helping to lower stress and ease the load on your digestive system. Both practices are accessible and can be tailored to fit even the busiest schedules, offering a respite in the midst of life's chaos.

- Social support can go a long way in managing stress and should not be overlooked. Humans are inherently social beings, and relationships can be a source of immense strength and comfort. Building a supportive network—whether through family, friends, or community groups—provides a buffer against stress. Engaging in group activities or clubs not only fosters connection but also offers a shared sense of purpose and belonging. These connections can provide a listening ear, a shoulder to lean on, or simply a distraction from daily pressures. By nurturing these relationships, you create a safety net of support that can ease the burdens of stress, allowing your gut to heal and thrive.

- Meditation: Consider setting aside time for regular meditation sessions. These moments of mindfulness can ground you, helping to center your thoughts and calm your body.

- Setting boundaries is a powerful way to manage your workload and protect your mental health. By clearly delineating your personal and professional time, you can prevent burnout and preserve your energy for what truly matters.

These strategies are not about eliminating stress but rather managing it in a way that supports your gut health and overall well-being. Integrating stress management into your daily life doesn't have to be complicated. Simple practices can weave seamlessly into your routine, offering relief without requiring drastic changes.

The Role of Physical Activity in Digestion

Picture a winding river, flowing effortlessly through valleys and plains, carrying with it life and nutrients. This is much like your digestive tract when you engage in regular physical activity. Exercise is not merely a means to maintain your physical appearance; it plays a crucial role in keeping your digestive system functioning smoothly.

Regular movement enhances gut motility, which is the speed at which food travels through your intestines. When you exercise, your body increases the production of hormones that stimulate peristalsis, the rhythmic contractions of the intestinal muscles. This process helps prevent constipation and ensures that food moves efficiently through your digestive tract, much like that river carrying life downstream. Additionally, exercise influences the composition of your gut microbiome, promoting a diverse and balanced community of bacteria. This diversity is linked to improved digestion, better nutrient absorption, and a stronger immune system, underscoring the profound impact of physical activity on your gut health.

When considering specific exercises to support digestion, walking stands out as an accessible and effective option. It may seem simple, but a brisk walk can do wonders for your digestive health. The gentle motion stimulates the muscles in your abdomen, promoting regular bowel movements and reducing bloating. It's a low-impact activity that can be easily incorporated into your daily routine, whether it's a stroll around the block or a walk after dinner.

Yoga is another excellent choice, offering a holistic approach that combines physical movement with mindfulness. Certain yoga poses, such as twists and forward folds, massage and stimulate your internal organs, enhancing digestion and alleviating discomfort.

For those seeking a more vigorous workout, high-intensity interval training (HIIT) can be beneficial. HIIT boosts metabolic rate and promotes fat loss, indirectly supporting gut health by reducing inflammation and improving insulin sensitivity. Whatever your preference, incorporating these activities into your lifestyle can lead to significant improvements in your digestive health.

While exercise is beneficial, balance and moderation are key. Over-exercising, particularly through excessive endurance training, can have the opposite effect, placing undue stress on your body and digestive system. Intense, prolonged workouts without adequate recovery can lead to increased cortisol levels, a stress hormone that can negatively impact gut health. This can result in symptoms like bloating, cramping, and changes in bowel habits, which can be discouraging.

It's important to listen to your body and recognize the signs when you're pushing too hard. Rest and recovery days are not just a luxury; they are essential for allowing your body to repair and strengthen. By balancing your exercise routine with adequate rest, you provide your gut with the environment it needs to thrive.

Integrating physical activity into your daily routine doesn't have to be daunting.

- Start by setting realistic fitness goals that align with your lifestyle and preferences. Whether it's committing to a certain number of steps each day or attending a weekly yoga class, having clear goals can help keep you motivated.

- Creating a varied workout schedule can also keep things interesting and prevent burnout. Mix different types of exercises, such as cardio, strength training, and flexibility work, to engage different muscle groups and support overall health.

- Remember, consistency is more important than intensity. Even short bursts of activity can make a difference, so find what works for you and stick with it.

Mindfulness and the Gut: Practicing Intuitive Eating

Intuitive eating is about reconnecting with your body's natural signals, particularly those of hunger and fullness. It's a philosophy that encourages you to trust your internal cues rather than external diet rules. By listening to your body, you honor its needs, eating when you're truly hungry and stopping when you're satisfied. This approach helps you avoid emotional eating, where stress or boredom rather than hunger drive food choices. It supports your gut by reducing the digestive stress caused by overeating or eating when not truly hungry. When you eat intuitively, you foster a healthier relationship with food, one that is free from guilt and anxiety, allowing your digestive system to function more efficiently.

Mindfulness, being fully present in the moment, profoundly impacts digestion. When you engage in mindful eating, you slow down and savor each bite, enhancing the sensory experience of eating. This practice allows you to appreciate the flavors, textures, and aromas of your food, making meals more satisfying. By focusing on your meal, you can improve digestive efficiency, as the body is not overwhelmed or distracted. Mindfulness also encourages you to chew thoroughly, aiding in the mechanical breakdown of food and easing the burden on your stomach. This mindful approach to eating can lead to better nutrient absorption and a reduction in digestive discomfort, as the body can process food more effectively.

Implementing intuitive eating requires a shift in mindset and practice. One effective technique is keeping a food and feelings journal, where you document not only what you eat but how you feel before and after meals. This practice can help you identify patterns, such as emotional triggers for eating or foods that cause discomfort. Writing down your observations encourages reflection, helping you become more attuned to your body's signals. Practicing gratitude before meals is another powerful tool. By taking a moment to appreciate the food before you, you create a positive, mindful space that enhances the eating experience. This simple act can transform meals into moments of nourishment and connection, rather than mere consumption.

Transitioning to intuitive eating can pose challenges, particularly if you've been entrenched in diet culture's rigid rules. Overcoming the diet mentality involves letting go of the notion that foods are 'good' or 'bad.' Instead, focus on how foods make you feel and their effects on your body. Building trust with your internal cues takes time, especially if you've ignored them for years. Start by paying attention to the subtle signs of hunger and fullness, allowing yourself to respond naturally. It may feel uncomfortable initially, but with practice, you'll learn to trust your body's wisdom. This journey is not about perfection but progress, finding balance and peace with food.

Reflect on your current relationship with food. Are you eating out of habit, stress, or boredom, or responding to your body's true needs? Consider how mindfulness and intuitive eating could transform your digestive health and overall well-being. By embracing these practices, you cultivate a compassionate and respectful relationship with your body, supporting its natural rhythms and promoting a harmonious digestive system. This approach nurtures not just your gut but your entire being, creating a foundation for a healthier, more fulfilled life.

Digital Detox: Limiting Screen Time for Better Sleep

Consider the evening hours, a time when the world should be winding down, signaling our bodies to rest and rejuvenate. Yet, the reality is that the world never stops, and for many, this period is illuminated by the persistent glow of screens—smartphones, tablets, and televisions—keeping us tethered to the digital world. This constant exposure, particularly to blue light emitted by these devices, can significantly disrupt our sleep patterns. Blue light interferes with melatonin production, the hormone responsible for regulating sleep-wake cycles. As melatonin levels drop, falling asleep becomes a challenge, leading to restless nights and sluggish days. This disruption doesn't just affect sleep; it extends to your digestive health, as the body's rhythms become misaligned, impacting everything from digestion to nutrient absorption.

Engaging in late-night screen time can lead to a cascade of digestive issues. The artificial light and mental stimulation from screens can delay bedtime, resulting in irregular eating patterns and late-night snacking. This habit can burden your digestive system, which is naturally less active at night, causing discomfort and poor digestion. The impact is compounded by stress and anxiety levels, which often rise with increased screen time, further aggravating gut health. By understanding the intricate connection between digital device use and your body's natural processes, you can begin to appreciate the importance of setting boundaries for screen time, particularly in the hours leading up to bedtime.

Embarking on a digital detox can be a transformative step toward enhancing your overall well-being. By consciously reducing screen time, you create space for improved sleep quality and duration. This change not only restores your body's natural rhythms but also alleviates stress and anxiety, offering a reprieve from the constant barrage of digital stimuli.

Without the distraction of screens, your mind is free to unwind, allowing for deeper, more restorative sleep. This restfulness extends to your physical health, supporting processes like digestion and immune function, which are closely linked to adequate sleep. By prioritizing a digital detox, you take an active role in balancing your mental and physical health, cultivating a more harmonious lifestyle.

We've discussed this in part, but it's important to reiterate the detrimental effects electronic devices can have on sleep.

To initiate a digital detox:

- Consider establishing screen-free zones in your home. Designate areas like the bedroom or dining room as technology-free sanctuaries, encouraging relaxation and connection with loved ones.

- Setting specific times for digital breaks can also help you manage screen time more effectively. Choose periods during the day to step away from devices, allowing yourself to engage in offline activities that bring joy and fulfillment. These breaks not only reduce screen exposure but also foster mindfulness, helping you reconnect with yourself and the present moment.

By incorporating these practices into your routine, you create an environment conducive to digital balance and overall wellness.

Maintaining a healthy relationship with technology doesn't mean eliminating it entirely but rather using it mindfully and intentionally.

- Schedule regular tech-free activities, such as reading, drawing, or outdoor pursuits, to encourage a life beyond the screen. These activities can provide a much-needed reset, nurturing your creativity and well-being.

- Additionally, consider using apps designed to monitor and manage screen time. These tools can offer insights into your digital habits, helping you set limits and make informed choices about screen use.

By approaching technology with awareness and balance, you can integrate it into your life in a way that supports rather than detracts from your health and happiness.

Breathing Techniques to Enhance Gut Function

Breathing is something we do without thinking, yet its impact on our health is profound, particularly when it comes to digestion. The simple act of breathing can activate the parasympathetic nervous system, often referred to as the "rest and digest" system. This part of our nervous system encourages relaxation and supports the digestive process.

When you take slow, deep breaths, you enhance blood flow to your digestive organs, ensuring they receive the oxygen and nutrients they need to function optimally. This increased circulation can soothe your gut, reduce inflammation, and improve nutrient absorption, creating a more harmonious digestive environment. Proper breathing can also help manage stress, a common culprit of digestive disorders. By calming your mind, you indirectly support your gut health, reducing symptoms of conditions like IBS and promoting overall well-being.

Various breathing exercises can be particularly beneficial for digestive health. **Diaphragmatic breathing**, also known as belly breathing, is a technique that emphasizes deep breaths from the diaphragm rather than shallow breaths from the chest. This method can help relax the gastrointestinal tract and reduce tension.

To practice:

- Sit or lie down in a comfortable position.

- Place one hand on your chest and the other on your belly.

- Inhale deeply through your nose, allowing your belly to rise, then slowly exhale through your mouth.

- Repeat this process for several minutes, focusing on the rise and fall of your belly.

Alternate nostril breathing is another effective technique that promotes balance within the body. It involves inhaling and exhaling through one nostril while closing the other with a finger, then switching sides. This exercise can help calm the mind and body, facilitating better digestion and stress reduction.

Incorporating these breathing exercises into your daily routine is straightforward. Start with guided deep breathing sessions, setting aside a few minutes each day to focus on your breath. Consider integrating these exercises into your morning or evening routine, using them as a way to center yourself. Over time, these practices can become second nature, providing a reliable method for managing stress and supporting digestive health. Breathwork can also be integrated into meditation practices, enhancing the calming effects and deepening your sense of awareness. Breath-focused yoga classes offer another opportunity to explore the connection between breath and body, promoting relaxation and digestive harmony.

Regular practice of breathwork can lead to long-term improvements in digestion. By continuously engaging the parasympathetic nervous system, you train your body to respond more effectively to stressors, reducing their impact on your gut. This resilience can lead to fewer digestive disruptions and a more balanced gut environment. The benefits of breathwork extend beyond the gut, promoting overall mental clarity and emotional stability. As you continue to cultivate this practice, you may find that your relationship with your body deepens, fostering a greater sense of connection and understanding.

(For more in-depth instruction on proper breathing for health and relaxation, see Appendix I: Learning to Breathe)

CHAPTER 9
IMPLEMENTING CHANGES AND SUSTAINING SUCCESS

Building a Support System for Gut Health

Have you ever noticed how much easier it is to stick to a new habit when you have someone cheering you on? There's something profoundly comforting about knowing you're not alone, especially when embarking on a journey toward better health. This is where the power of a supportive network comes into play. Imagine a team of allies, each contributing a unique piece to your wellness puzzle. They offer encouragement, share wisdom, and sometimes, challenge you to push a little further than you thought possible. Social support is not just a nice-to-have; it's a cornerstone of sustainable health transformation.

Families hold a unique power to shape health habits. Picture a dinner table where each family member contributes to meal preparation, making choices together that nourish the body and the soul, then discussing their choices and future meal possibilities, sharing knowledge and joy.

Family involvement in dietary changes can transform a single-person initiative into a shared journey, creating an environment where healthy choices become the norm. When parents model balanced eating and involve children in meal planning, they instill lifelong habits. Children learn the value of nutrition, and the family as a unit becomes stronger, more cohesive. This shared responsibility fosters an atmosphere of mutual support, where everyone's health goals are respected and encouraged.

Friends, too, play a crucial role as accountability partners. They provide camaraderie and motivation, making the path to wellness less daunting. Whether it's a weekly yoga class or a commitment to try a new recipe together, having friends by your side can make all the difference. They celebrate your victories, no matter how small, and offer a listening ear when challenges arise. This companionship can be a powerful motivator, helping you stay committed to your goals even when the journey gets tough. By surrounding yourself with positive influences, you create a support system that bolsters your resolve and keeps you moving forward.

Within this support network, certain key figures can lend their expertise and insight. Nutritionists and dietitians offer invaluable guidance, helping you tailor your dietary choices to meet your unique needs. Their expertise can help you navigate the often-confusing world of nutrition, providing clarity and direction. Online support groups, too, can be a treasure trove of shared experiences and encouragement. These communities connect you with others on similar paths, offering a platform to exchange tips, discuss challenges, and celebrate successes. The sense of belonging that comes from being part of a community can be a powerful force for change, reinforcing your commitment to health.

Creating and maintaining a supportive environment requires intentional effort. Consider hosting regular meal prep sessions with friends, where you can experiment with new recipes, share cooking tips, and enjoy each other's company. These gatherings not only foster a sense of community but also make healthy eating more enjoyable and sustainable. Joining local wellness clubs or groups can also provide opportunities to connect with like-minded individuals, offering both social engagement and motivation. These clubs often host events, workshops, and activities that keep you inspired and informed, providing a steady stream of encouragement and support.

Communication is the glue that holds any support system together. Openly sharing your progress, challenges, and goals with loved ones fosters trust and understanding. This transparency invites feedback, allowing others to offer constructive insights and encouragement. It also strengthens relationships, as those around you feel more invested in your journey. By engaging in honest conversations, you create a space where everyone feels heard and valued, enhancing the sense of community and mutual support. Whether it's a family member, friend, or mentor, having someone to share your journey with can make all the difference.

Interactive Element: Establish a Support Network Map

Create a support network map, identifying individuals and groups that can assist in your health journey. Include family, friends, professionals, and online communities. Reflect on how each contributes to your goals and consider reaching out to strengthen these connections. Use this map to remind yourself of the resources available to you, ensuring you remain supported and motivated.

1. Begin by drawing a circle on a large piece of paper or posterboard. Write: "Social Network" inside the circle.
2. From there, draw lines to smaller circles titled: Friends, Family, Associates, Social Media Connections, Coworkers, Professionals, or anyone else you want to add.
3. From each of these circles, draw another line and circle with the names of individual people in each. Write their relationship to you and how they can contribute to your goals in this journey.

This can be fairly simple and limited or elaborate and extensive. It's a great way to see the overall picture of who might influence or help you and how. I prefer the tactile presence of paper, but you can also use an **app** to do this.

You can also use mapping like this to keep track of food and symptoms. Simply write: Journal in the center circle. Your first-row extensions would be the foods you eat, one for each circle. From there, your circle extensions would be symptoms, times, and other results of eating that food. (See 9,2 Staying Motivated)

Staying Motivated: Tracking Your Progress

In the whirlwind of daily life, it's easy to lose sight of your health goals. This is where tracking comes in as a powerful ally. Monitoring your progress serves as a constant reminder of your commitment to gut health, anchoring your efforts with tangible evidence of change. Imagine flipping through a journal filled with notes on dietary shifts you've made or symptoms you've conquered. Each entry becomes a testament to your dedication, a visual narrative of your journey. By recording changes and outcomes, you not only keep track of what works but also identify patterns and triggers, making it easier to adjust your approach as needed. This kind of documentation transforms abstract goals into concrete steps, boosting your motivation to stay the course.

Today's technology offers a myriad of tools to simplify tracking. Apps designed for food intake and symptom monitoring let you log meals and reactions with ease, providing instant feedback on how your gut responds to different foods. Wearable devices can monitor physical activity, sleep quality, and even stress levels, offering insights into how these factors interplay with your digestive health. These digital companions provide a comprehensive view of your lifestyle, helping you make informed decisions. By utilizing these tools, you create a personalized database that empowers you to track your journey with precision and clarity, ensuring that you stay informed and motivated.

Setting goals that are both realistic and achievable is crucial in maintaining momentum. Breaking down larger objectives into smaller, manageable steps can make them feel less overwhelming. Instead of aiming to overhaul your entire diet, start by introducing one new gut-friendly food each week. This approach allows you to celebrate small successes, which can be incredibly motivating. Recognize each milestone, no matter how minor it may seem. Whether it's a week without digestive discomfort or the successful introduction of a new fiber-rich food, these victories deserve acknowledgment. Celebrating these moments reinforces your efforts, fostering a positive cycle of achievement and motivation.

Tracking progress also offers profound psychological benefits. There's something deeply satisfying about seeing your journey laid out in charts and graphs, each data point representing a step closer to your goals. Visualizing progress can boost your confidence, confirming that your efforts are yielding results. Reflecting on past challenges you've overcome can provide a sense of achievement and resilience, reminding you of your capability to tackle obstacles. This reflection not only builds self-assurance but also strengthens your resolve to continue pursuing your health objectives. By acknowledging how far you've come, you fortify your commitment to forging ahead, armed with the knowledge and experience you've gained.

Visual Element: Progress Chart

Create a chart to visualize your progress, marking milestones, dietary changes, and symptom improvements. Use this chart as a motivational tool, celebrating each achievement and identifying areas for further focus. This visual representation serves as a daily reminder of your journey, keeping you inspired and engaged in your health pursuits.

Overcoming Setbacks: What to Do When Symptoms Persist

Navigating the path to better health is rarely a straight line. Setbacks, though often frustrating, are a natural part of the process. Imagine them as the unexpected detours on a road trip—unwelcome, but not insurmountable. Recognizing that these moments will happen allows you to approach them with patience and resilience. Common triggers for setbacks include dietary changes, stress, or even environmental factors like travel or illness. Chronic conditions, such as irritable bowel syndrome or food sensitivities, may mean that symptoms ebb and flow despite your best efforts. Accepting this reality can shift your perspective, transforming setbacks from roadblocks to opportunities for learning and adjustment.

When symptoms persist, it's crucial to reassess and adapt your strategies. Start by revisiting your dietary plan. Consider keeping a detailed food diary to identify any patterns or specific foods that might be contributing to your discomfort. Sometimes, a minor tweak—like adjusting fiber intake or introducing a new probiotic—can make a world of difference. Consulting healthcare professionals can provide fresh insights and guidance. They might suggest tests to identify new triggers or recommend therapies you haven't yet explored. Their expertise can often illuminate pathways you might not have considered, providing renewed hope and direction.

Resilience and persistence become your strongest allies when facing ongoing challenges. The ability to bounce back and learn from setbacks is what propels you forward. Each setback offers a chance to refine your approach, enhancing your understanding of your body's unique needs. Maintaining a positive outlook, even in the face of discomfort, can have a profound impact on your journey. Remember that progress is not always linear and that each step, no matter how small, brings you closer to your goals.

Cultivating a mindset that embraces growth and change allows you to navigate obstacles with grace and determination, fostering resilience that transcends gut health.

For those moments when you feel stuck, knowing where to turn for additional support can be invaluable. Seeking specialist consultations can provide deeper insights into your condition, helping you uncover underlying issues that may be contributing to persistent symptoms. Specialists can offer tailored advice and treatments, aligning with your specific needs and goals. Online forums and support groups can also be a rich resource for advice and encouragement. Connecting with others who share similar experiences can offer not only practical tips but also a sense of camaraderie. These communities provide a platform to share stories, exchange ideas, and draw strength from collective wisdom.

Textual Element: Resource List for Persistent Symptoms

Create a resource list that includes contact information for specialists, recommended books, and online support groups. This list will serve as a go-to guide when seeking further assistance, ensuring you have access to the support and information you need to address ongoing challenges. This tool empowers you to take proactive steps toward resolving persistent issues, fostering a sense of agency and confidence in your health journey.

Celebrating Small Wins in Gut Health

In the pursuit of better gut health, it's crucial to recognize and celebrate the small victories along the way. These incremental achievements are the building blocks of long-term success. When you successfully manage a week without digestive discomfort or notice improved energy levels from dietary changes, these aren't just minor victories; they are significant milestones that deserve acknowledgment. Recognizing these wins helps to maintain motivation and satisfaction, reinforcing the positive behaviors that led to them. It can be as simple as feeling less bloated after meals or sticking to your meal plan consistently for a month. Each small step forward is a reminder of your progress, helping to keep the momentum going even when the journey feels challenging.

Celebrating these achievements provides an opportunity to appreciate your efforts and resilience. Treating yourself to a special activity or experience as a reward can be a powerful motivator. Perhaps you indulge in a relaxing day at a spa, a new book, or an invigorating outdoor adventure. These rewards not only celebrate your hard work but also serve as a reminder of why you embarked on this path in the first place. Sharing your successes with a supportive community can amplify the joy of these moments. Whether it's posting about your progress on social media or discussing it with a friend, celebrating with others can reinforce your commitment and inspire those around you.

Positive reinforcement plays a crucial role in habit formation and self-confidence. When you acknowledge your progress, you reinforce the behaviors that contributed to it, making them more likely to become ingrained habits. This strengthening of self-efficacy—the belief in your ability to succeed—can have a profound impact on your overall mindset. It's the reason why you might feel a surge of pride after sticking to your goals, even when the going gets tough. By celebrating your accomplishments, you create a positive feedback loop that encourages continued effort and growth, making it easier to tackle future challenges.

Setting new goals after achieving milestones is vital for maintaining momentum. These goals keep the journey dynamic and exciting, allowing you to continue pushing your boundaries. After achieving a dietary consistency goal, you might set your sights on increasing your physical activity or exploring new gut-friendly foods. Each new challenge provides an opportunity for growth and learning, encouraging you to expand your horizons and deepen your understanding of your body's needs. Reflecting on past successes can be a great source of inspiration for setting these new goals. Remembering how far you've come not only boosts your confidence but also provides valuable insights into what strategies worked well for you. This reflection helps you build on your strengths and address areas where you might need to adapt your approach.

Engaging with the Gut Health Community

Connecting with others who share your health goals can be a transformative experience. Involvement in a community offers a wealth of support, knowledge, and inspiration. By engaging with others who are also focused on improving their gut health, you gain access to shared experiences and insights that can accelerate your progress. The collective wisdom of a community can provide solutions to challenges you may face, offering new perspectives and ideas that you might not have considered. This sense of belonging and shared purpose can be incredibly motivating, reinforcing your commitment to your health goals and providing a buffer against setbacks.

There are numerous platforms where you can engage with the gut health community. Online forums and social media groups offer a convenient way to connect with others, share your experiences, and seek advice. These digital spaces provide a platform for exchanging tips, discussing the latest research, and celebrating successes together. Local health workshops and events offer opportunities for face-to-face interaction, allowing you to build relationships and learn from experts in the field. These gatherings can be a great source of motivation and inspiration, providing a sense of camaraderie and support that can be invaluable on your health journey.

Active participation in community activities can enhance your experience and deepen your engagement. Sharing your personal experiences and insights can provide valuable contributions to the community, helping others learn from your journey. Attending webinars and discussion panels can expand your knowledge and keep you informed about the latest developments in gut health. These interactions not only enrich your understanding but also foster a sense of empowerment, as you take an active role in your health journey and contribute to the collective knowledge of the community. Engaging with the community in this way can provide a continuous source of motivation and support, helping you stay committed to your goals and inspiring others to do the same.

Being part of a community also helps you stay informed about the latest research and trends in gut health. Access to expert advice through community connections can provide valuable insights and guidance, helping you make informed decisions about your health. Learning about new studies and findings keeps you up-to-date with advancements in the field, ensuring that your strategies remain aligned with the latest evidence. This knowledge empowers you to adapt your approach as needed, ensuring that your health journey is guided by the best available information. The community serves as a valuable resource, providing a wealth of information and support to help you achieve your health goals.

The journey toward optimal gut health is enriched immeasurably by community involvement. Whether it's a tip shared about a new probiotic or a success story about overcoming a particularly stubborn digestive issue, the exchange of knowledge and experiences injects motivation into your own efforts.

Being part of a community also plays a crucial role in staying informed about the latest gut health research and trends. Access to expert advice through community connections can provide valuable insights and guidance, helping you make informed decisions about your health journey. Learning about new studies and findings keeps you up-to-date with advancements in the field, ensuring that your strategies remain aligned with the latest evidence.

Community achievements act as a powerful motivator, showing what's possible and igniting the drive to push through challenges.

There are various platforms where you can engage with the gut health community. Online forums and social media groups are accessible spaces where individuals from all walks of life come together to discuss their health journeys. These digital platforms provide an opportunity to connect with others in real-time, sharing insights and advice across distances. Whether you're seeking a quick recipe swap or in-depth discussions on the latest gut health trends, these forums are vibrant hubs of interaction.

Local health workshops and events offer face-to-face engagement, allowing for deeper connections and direct learning experiences. These gatherings often feature experts who provide valuable insights and facilitate discussions, creating environments where learning and networking flourish. By participating in these workshops, you gain access to a wealth of information and form meaningful bonds with others on similar paths.

Actively participating in community activities can significantly enrich your experience and bolster your commitment to gut health. Sharing your personal experiences and insights allows you to contribute to the collective knowledge, helping others learn from your journey while reinforcing your own understanding. Attending webinars and discussion panels offers opportunities to expand your knowledge and stay informed about the latest developments in the field. These events often feature experts who share cutting-edge research and practical advice, equipping you with the tools to make informed decisions about your health. By engaging with these resources, you not only deepen your own understanding but also inspire others through your active involvement.

The community serves as a valuable resource, providing a wealth of information and support to help you achieve your health goals. This shared knowledge fosters a sense of empowerment, as you navigate your journey with the confidence that comes from being informed and supported by a network of like-minded individuals.

The Future of Gut Health: Embracing Science and Technology

Imagine standing on the brink of a new era in understanding gut health, where science and technology merge to unlock possibilities, we couldn't have fathomed just a few years ago. Advances in microbiome sequencing technologies are at the forefront of this transformation, offering insights into the intricate ecosystem within us. With these tools, we can now map the vast diversity of microbes living in our digestive tracts, understanding not just their presence but their function and interaction with our bodies. This detailed view allows researchers to identify specific microbial signatures associated with health and disease, paving the way for targeted interventions that could redefine how we approach gut-related conditions.

The gut-brain axis, once a mystery, is being illuminated by cutting-edge research revealing profound connections between our digestive and nervous systems. New insights show how gut microbes influence brain function, affecting everything from mood to cognitive abilities. This burgeoning field of study holds promise for developing therapies that address mental health challenges through gut health, offering new hope for those struggling with conditions like anxiety and depression. As our understanding deepens, the potential for personalized treatments grows, moving us closer to a future where gut health is integral to mental wellness strategies.

Technology is also enhancing how we manage and personalize gut health strategies. Artificial intelligence is being harnessed to provide personalized nutrition recommendations based on individual microbiome profiles. This means that dietary advice can be tailored with unprecedented precision, ensuring that each person receives guidance that aligns with their unique biological makeup. Apps that track microbiome changes and health data are becoming increasingly sophisticated, allowing users to monitor their gut health in real-time.

These digital tools offer insights into how lifestyle choices impact the microbiome, empowering you to make informed decisions and adapt your habits to optimize gut health.

Innovative treatments and interventions are emerging as well, reshaping the landscape of gut health care. Fecal microbiota transplantation (FMT) is gaining traction as a groundbreaking therapy for restoring healthy gut flora, especially in cases where traditional treatments fall short. This procedure involves transferring stool from a healthy donor to a patient, introducing beneficial bacteria that can rebalance the gut ecosystem. The development of targeted prebiotics and probiotics is another exciting frontier. These specialized supplements are designed to nourish specific beneficial bacteria or introduce new strains, tailored to address individual health needs.

Staying informed and adaptable in this rapidly evolving field is crucial. As scientific progress continues, being open to new approaches will allow you to make the most of emerging therapies and technologies. Following reputable health sources and publications can keep you updated on the latest research and findings. This ongoing education will enable you to refine your health strategies, ensuring they remain aligned with the latest evidence-based insights. Being adaptable means being willing to adjust your approach as new information becomes available, embracing change as an opportunity for growth and improved health.

The chapter concludes with a gentle reminder that the journey of optimizing gut health is one of continuous learning. The integration of science and technology opens new doors, offering possibilities that were once beyond our reach. As you explore these advancements, you're not just investing in your health today but laying the groundwork for a future where gut health is a cornerstone of overall wellness. This journey is personal yet interconnected with the broader landscape of human health, and as you move forward, remember that every step you take contributes to a deeper understanding and appreciation of the incredible ecosystem within you.

CONCLUSION

As we come to the end of our journey together, I want to take a moment to reflect on the incredible power of gut health. Throughout this book, we've explored the intricate connection between our digestive system and every aspect of our well-being. We've seen how the trillions of microbes that reside within us play a pivotal role in shaping our physical, mental, and emotional health. By nurturing this inner ecosystem, we unlock the potential for a happier, more vibrant life.

Let's recap the key points we've covered.

- We began by understanding the gut's ecosystem, the delicate balance of bacteria that influences digestion, immunity, and even our mood.

- We explored the gut-brain connection, discovering how the health of our digestive system impacts our mental well-being.

- We delved into common digestive disorders and learned strategies for managing them through diet and lifestyle changes.

- We also traced the importance of gut health across the lifespan, from nurturing children's microbiomes to supporting digestive function as we age.

- We discovered the cornerstone of gut health: nutrition. By focusing on probiotic-rich foods, prebiotic fibers, and a balanced, anti-inflammatory diet, we learned how to cultivate a thriving gut garden.

- We explored the profound impact of lifestyle factors like sleep, stress management, and physical activity on our digestive health.

Throughout this journey, I've shared actionable insights and transformative strategies.

- By incorporating fermented foods, practicing mindful eating, and prioritizing sleep, you can begin to reshape your gut health today.

- Engaging in stress-reduction techniques like deep breathing and embracing the power of a digital detox can have a profound impact on your digestive well-being. Remember, small changes can yield significant results.

But this is just the beginning. I invite you to take charge of your gut health journey, to become the architect of your own wellness.

- Start by implementing the 4-week gut healing protocol outlined in this book.
- Keep a food and symptom journal to track your progress and celebrate your successes along the way.

- Embrace the power of personalization, tailoring your approach to your unique needs and goals.

You don't have to walk this path alone. Join our vibrant community of gut health enthusiasts, where you can find support, inspiration, and a wealth of shared experiences. Engage with others who are on a similar journey, exchange recipes and tips, and celebrate each other's victories. Together, we can create a movement that prioritizes gut health as the foundation for a happier, healthier life.

As we look to the future, I am filled with hope and excitement. The field of gut health is rapidly evolving, with new research and technologies emerging every day. By staying informed and adaptable, we can harness these advancements to optimize our digestive well-being. The possibilities are endless, and I am confident that together, we can create a world where gut health is at the forefront of our approach to wellness.

So, my dear reader, I leave you with this final thought:

Your gut is your gateway to a life filled with vitality, resilience, and joy. Cherish it, nourish it, and listen to its wisdom. You have the power within you to transform your health and your life. Embrace this journey with curiosity, compassion, and an open heart. The path to a happier, healthier you begins in the gut, and I am honored to have been a part of your journey.

APPENDIX I: LEARNING TO BREATHE

For most of us, breathing has become an incomplete, superficial and sometimes hasty procedure. The action of breathing is a powerful driving force in circulation. It moves oxygen deeply through the bloodstream. If you have a sedentary job or lifestyle, you've likely developed congestion in one organ or another. With complete breathing, the bloodstream in organs is prevented from slowing down to the point where it stagnates and degenerates from "stream" to "marsh".

When you breathe in, blood is moved through every tissue in the body. The optimum interchange of gases in the lungs—the absorption of oxygen and the giving off of carbon dioxide—is at its most efficient when breathing is deep, complete and slow. The large vein continuously pouring blood from the liver into the heart is emptied regularly through suction developed by the lungs in breathing. When the venous blood from the liver can't circulate freely, it becomes congested and causes repercussions throughout the body.

It's best to practice breathing lying down.

- First remove any article of clothing or jewelry that will constrict your neck, chest, lungs, belly, or diaphragm.

- Lie on your back on a firm surface (not your bed).

- Legs should be straight and arms comfortably down along your sides, palms up and elbows gently tucked near the waist.

- Tuck your shoulder blades under to lift your chest a bit and open up your rib cage.

- Do not arch the neck or tuck the head or chin. Your head should be in a natural position with chin pointed toward the opposite wall.

- If necessary, place a low soft pillow under your knees to diminish the lumbar arch.

- Closing your eyes will help you concentrate.

- Relax all the organs and muscles designed to hold things in or hold you up.

1. Exhale first through your nose.

    - Until a receptacle is empty, it cannot be filled, so in the act of respiration, a slow and complete exhalation is an absolute prerequisite of correct and complete inhalation.

    - Slowly and calmly exhale through your nose, forcing all air out of your lungs. The chest is depressed by its own weight, expelling air. This out-breath must be slow. At the end of the expiration, use your abdominal muscles to force remaining air out. To do this, pull your abdominal muscles inward, in a contraction toward your back to expel the last traces of tainted air. Because the spongy nature of the lungs does not allow them to fully empty, they will always retain some impure air. You're attempting to minimize that residue.

2. Breathe in through your nose.

    - Fill your lungs with air. Fill the diaphragm first, then the chest. You're not attempting to blow yourself up like a balloon. Breathe easily, slowly and silently. Think about the action of your lungs, rib cage, diaphragm, clavicle, and intestines as they rise and lower. You may need to yawn. This is a good sign, showing that your lungs are relaxed.

3. Hold inspiration (in-breath) for 5-20 seconds.

- When you breathe deeply, the surface of the tiny air sacs (alveoli) in your lungs is increased. All the normally inactive alveoli, unused in everyday breathing, are brought into service. When air remains in contact with lung alveoli, you receive the maximum degree of aeration.

4. Putting it all together.

- Lie on your back, exhale through your nose and then inhale through your nose. Begin breathing slowly and deeply from your diaphragm. When you feel that it's impossible to raise your diaphragm any more, expand your ribs and allow more air to enter your lungs. Once the ribs are fully extended, raise your collar bones so a little more air can enter. Remember, don't try to blow yourself up like a balloon. The whole process should be easy and comfortable.

- Avoid tensing your hands, face and neck.

- For this practice, hold the in-breath for 5-20 seconds and then slowly release air through the nose for a slow count of 5. When you reach 5, force the air from your lungs through the nose using the abdomen to press out any remaining air.

- Allow 2 short ordinary breaths before beginning again. Repeat 3 times.

There's a natural immunity attributed to the ionic balance in the blood that, in great part, depends on breathing. This exercise will teach you to focus on the diaphragm rather than primarily using the chest in shallow breathing, which is the way many people breathe on a daily basis. By learning to breathe properly, you'll learn to relax properly, and if you are not relaxed your body cannot digest food properly.

APPENDIX II:
LEARNING TO MEDITATE

Learning to meditate is another strategy to help you stay on track with anything you're trying to achieve.

Meditation is simply the act of focusing deeply, in silence, as a method of relaxing the mind so as to 'get in touch' with inner consciousness, thereby leading to self-discovery, self-renewal and spiritual growth.

You may wish to use meditation as a means of getting in touch with your own consciousness and how it plays a part in your behavior, the way you view yourself and your world. The patterns your mind has set up for you can more easily be changed when you learn to meditate deeply.

When you're deep in meditation, you have the opportunity to connect with that part of yourself that is overshadowed during daily waking hours, when everything is about time schedules and the hustle and bustle of everyday activities.

Learning to meditate is simple.

Choose a time when you can sit quietly for a designated period, when you will not be disturbed or distracted.

- Sit quietly in a relaxed position. Be sure you aren't so comfortable that you fall asleep! An upright chair works well, or you can sit on a mat or towel on the floor with your back straight.

- Cross your legs or extend them in a relaxed position. Your hands and arms can fall at your side or you can rest them on your thighs or knees with your palms facing up.

- Close your eyes and take a few deep breaths in and out through your nose. Try to breathe from the diaphragm not just the upper chest. Envision a place between your eyebrows. This is where the legendary 'third eye' is located. Focus on this spot.

- You might hear outside noises, such as a car passing. Let it pass and return your focus to your breathing. Give a visual component to your breath. Assign it a color and watch it move smoothly in through your nose, filling your lungs, and then moving freely out through your nose. (Blue is a good color to use because it represents peace and cooperation).

- As you begin to unwind, do not think about anything in particular. Your objective is to relax and 'see' the inner workings of your subconscious mind. Remain in the moment; don't let your mind wander.

The process of meditation follows a particular order. By following your breath, you will get into a rhythm that supports a relaxed mind. The mind is cleared, the body and mind are calmed, and the focus in inward, to the consciousness, not on the external world. When you reach a state of contemplation where you are no longer distracted by what's outside you, your meditation will deepen.

Meditation will enhance creativity and give you keener intuition, deeper sleep, heightened awareness, lower blood pressure, greater insight, and general well-being. With continued practice, you will start to see progressively greater results in your personal and professional life.

Isn't a good night's sleep as good as meditation?

When you're asleep, you're not consciously aware of what's going on around you. Only someone who is highly advanced can control their dreams in order to exact change or understand their meaning.

During meditation, you are conscious and awake, aware of your surroundings but able to 'tune them out'. You can, with enough practice, focus your subconscious mind on your cells, your physicality and your DNA, and in this way, you can potentially even heal your body.

Because of this heightened awareness, the subconscious takes its cue to make the change you are focused on, and in a short time, it will begin to carry over to your normal everyday state of mind. It will see this as a projection of what you are and will be reinforced each time you go deep into meditation.

You will be more aware about almost everything, and you will grow spiritually and personally.

Meditation is a great solution for people struggling with gut problems. Meditation can take you on a beautiful journey that will help you to live your life on your terms. It will take you out of your comfort zone and allow you to grow every single day while it reinforces only the good messages you put into your subconscious while you meditate.

Practicing meditation every day helps you learn how to listen to your body. When you meditate, the focus is on your inner self and not on the environment. Practice meditation every day for about 5-10 minutes or more if you can as a means of relaxing, learning about yourself and your behaviors, and retraining your subconscious to relay positive messages during your day. In this way, you can enjoy life more and be better able to serve those around you. You will realize that your goals are easily attainable through focused concentration, and you will be able to see that each task within your plan is simply part of who you were meant to be.

You will learn to love your path!

REFERENCES

"Your Digestive System and How it Works." National Institute of Diabetes and Digestive and Kidney Diseases. https://www.niddk.nih.gov/health-information/digestive-diseases/digestive-system-how-it-works. Accessed March 2025

Henkel, James S, Baldwin, Michael R., Barbieri, Joseph T. "Toxins from Bacteria." PubMed Central, National Library of Medicine. https://pmc.ncbi.nlm.nih.gov/articles/PMC3564551/ Accessed March 2025

Carmody, Rachel, PhD., Turnbaugh, Peter, PhD., et al. "Cooking Food Alters the Microbiome." University of California San Francisco. https://www.ucsf.edu/news/2019/09/415511/cooking-food-alters-microbiome Accessed March 2025

"What is the Vagus Nerve?" Cleveland Clinic. https://my.clevelandclinic.org/health/body/22279-vagus-nerve Accessed March 2025

Ruo-Gu Xiong, et al. "The Role of Gut Microbiota in Anxiety, Depressions, and Other Mental Disorders as Well as the Protective Effects of Dietary Components." PubMed Central. National Library of Medicine. https://pmc.ncbi.nlm.nih.gov/articles/PMC10384867/ Accessed March 2025

Merkouris, Ermis, et al. "Probiotics' Effects in the Treatment of Anxiety and Depression: A Comprehensive Review of 2014-2023 Clinical Trials." PubMed Central. National Library of Medicine. https://pmc.ncbi.nlm.nih.gov/articles/PMC10893170/#:~:text=Signif icant%20between%2Dgroup%20decrease%20in,found%20in%20the%20synbiotic%20group.&text=Students%20who%20consumed%20probiotics%2C%20showed,No%20adverse%20effects%20were%20noted. Accessed March 2025

Prasad, Chandan, et al. "Advanced Glycation End Products and Risks for Chronic Diseases: Intervening Through Lifestyle Modification." American Journal of Lifestyle Medicine. National Library of Medicine. https://pmc.ncbi.nlm.nih.gov/articles/PMC6600625/ Accessed March 2025

Levy, Jill. "Food Combining Benefits for Improved Digestion and Less Bloat." Ancient Nutrition. https://ancientnutrition.com/blogs/all/food-combining Accessed March 2025

Zhu, Huiyue, et al. " A psychobiotic approach to the treatment of depression: A systematic review and metasnalysis." Journal of Functional Foods. Science Direct. https://www.sciencedirect.com/science/article/pii/S175646462200069X#:~:text=In%20this%20study%2C%20fifteen%20RCTs,effect%20superior%20to%20the%20placebo. Accessed March 2025

Noor, Jawad, et al. "Exploring the Impact of the Gut Microbiome on Obesity and Weight Loss: A Review Article." Cureus. National Library of Medicine. https://pmc.ncbi.nlm.nih.gov/articles/PMC10368799/ Accessed March 2025

Ayesha, Ismat E., et al. "Probiotics and Their Role in the Management of Type 2 Diabetes Mellitus (Short-Term Versus Long-Term Effect): A Systematic Review and Meta-Analysis." Cureus. National Library of Medicine. https://pmc.ncbi.nlm.nih.gov/articles/PMC10631563/ Accessed March 2025

Lacy, Brian E., Patel, Nihal K. "Rome Criteria and a Diagnostic Approach to Irritable Bowel Syndrome." Journal of Clinical Medicine. National Library of Medicine. https://pmc.ncbi.nlm.nih.gov/articles/PMC5704116/ Accessed March 2025

"Low FODMAP Diet." Cleveland Clinic. https://my.clevelandclinic.org/health/treatments/22466-low-fodmap-diet Accessed March 2925

Paray, Bilal A., et al. "Leaky Gut and Autoimmunity: An Intricate Balance in Individuals Health and the Diseased State." International Journal of Molecular Sciences. National Library of Medicine. https://pmc.ncbi.nlm.nih.gov/articles/PMC7767453/ Accessed March 2025

"Probiotics: Fact Sheet for Health Professionals." Office of Dietary Supplements. National Institutes of Health. https://ods.od.nih.gov/factsheets/Probiotics-HealthProfessional/ Accessed March 2025

Leeuwendaal, Natasha, et al. "Fermented Foods, Health and the Gut Mirobiome." Nutrients. National Library of Medicine. https://pmc.ncbi.nlm.nih.gov/articles/PMC9003261/ Accessed March 2025

Eswaran, Shanti MD, FAC. "Low-FODMAP (Fermentable, Oligo-, Di-, Mono-saccharides, and Polyols) Diet." American College of Gastroenterology. https://gi.org/topics/low-fodmap-diet/ Accessed March 2025

Denhard, Morgan, MS, RD, LDN. "Digestive Enzymes and Digestive Enzyme Supplements." Health. Johns Hopkins Medicine. https://www.hopkinsmedicine.org/health/wellness-and-prevention/digestive-enzymes-and-digestive-enzyme-supplements#:~:text=Amylase%20(made%20in%20the%20mouth,the%20pancreas%3B%20breaks%20down%20proteins) Accessed March 2025

Printed in Dunstable, United Kingdom